ISBN-13: 978-1-63489-677-1
Library of Congress Control Number: 2023918078
Printed in the United States of America
First Printing: 2024
28 27 26 25 24 5 4 3 2 1

Illustrated by Katarina Stevanović
Cover and interior design by Aurora Whittet Best
Author photos by Hayley Volkmann

This book is typeset in OpenDyslexic, an open-sourced font created to increase readability for readers with dyslexia. Learn more at opendyslexic.org.

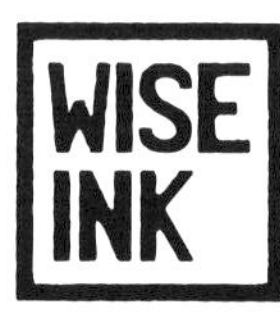

Wise Ink
PO Box 580195
Minneapolis, MN 55458-0195

Wise Ink is a creative publishing agency for game-changers. Wise Ink authors uplift, inspire, and inform, and their titles support building a better and more equitable world. For more information, visit wiseink.com.

To order, visit itascabooks.com or peycarter.com. Reseller discounts available.

Contact Pey Carter at peycarter.com for speaking engagements, freelance writing projects, and interviews.

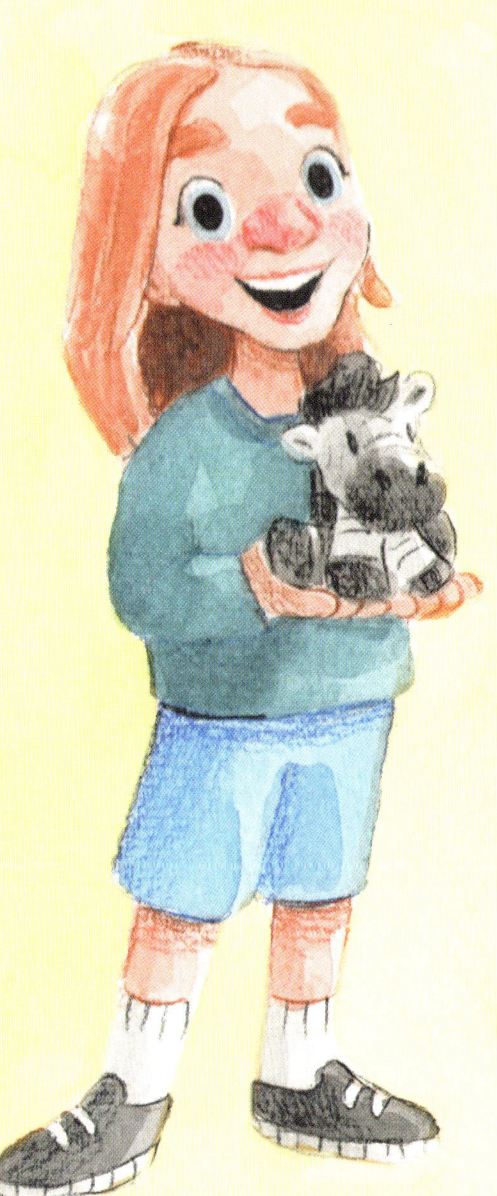

Bendy Bones and Stretchy Skin

An Ehlers-Danlos Book

Written by
Pey Carter & Abigail Bailey

Illustrated by
Katarina Stevanović

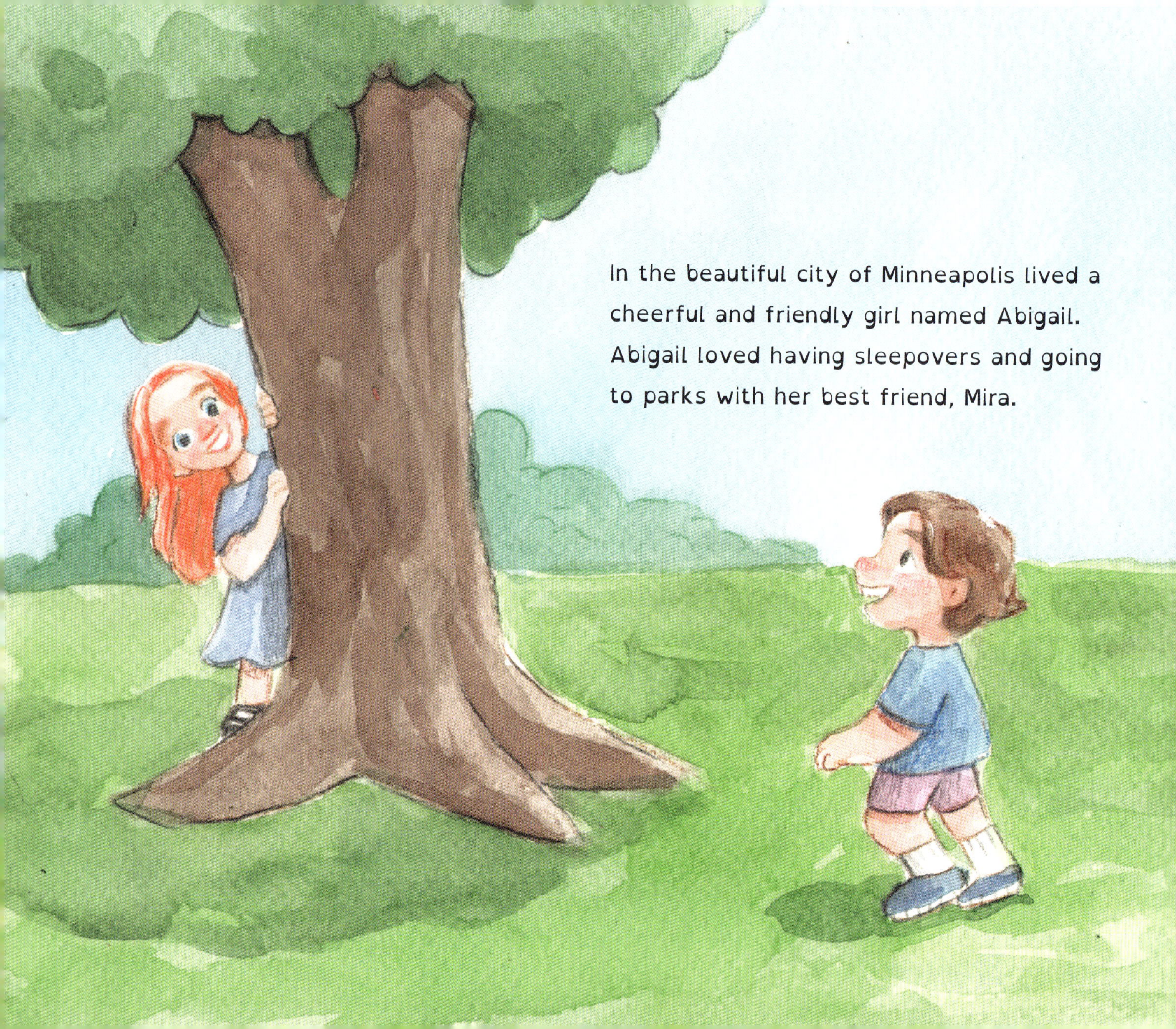

In the beautiful city of Minneapolis lived a cheerful and friendly girl named Abigail. Abigail loved having sleepovers and going to parks with her best friend, Mira.

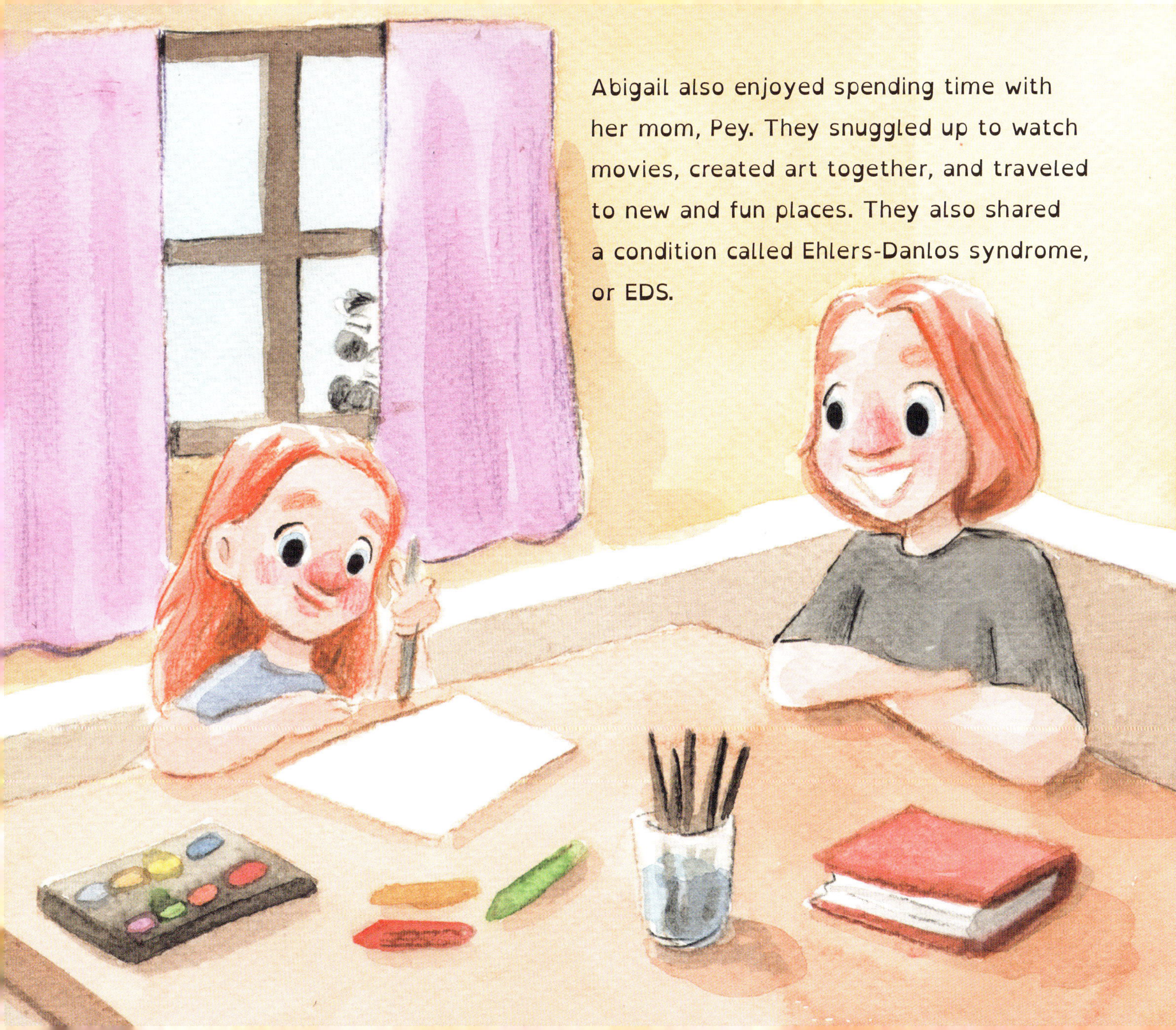

Abigail also enjoyed spending time with her mom, Pey. They snuggled up to watch movies, created art together, and traveled to new and fun places. They also shared a condition called Ehlers-Danlos syndrome, or EDS.

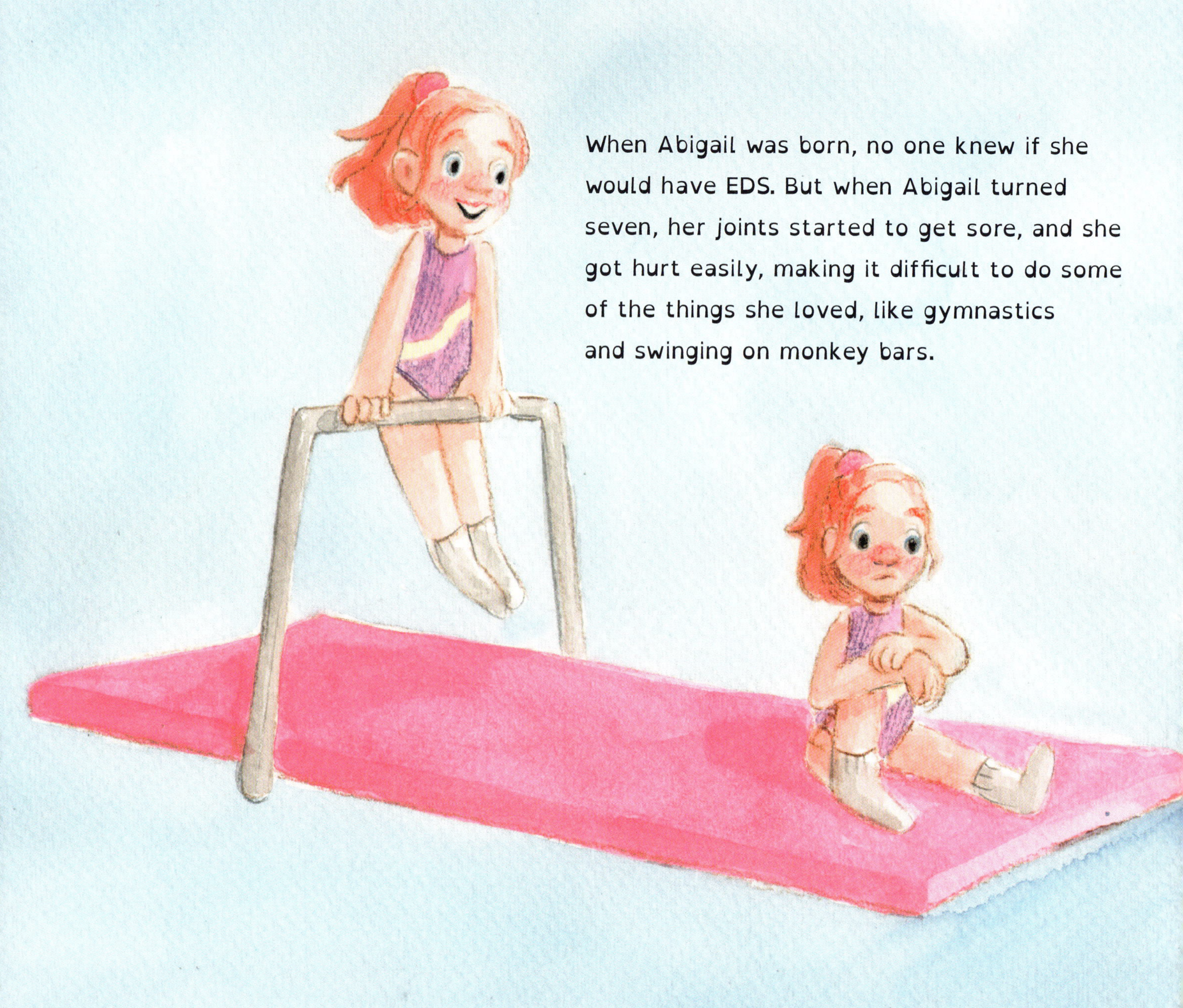

When Abigail was born, no one knew if she would have EDS. But when Abigail turned seven, her joints started to get sore, and she got hurt easily, making it difficult to do some of the things she loved, like gymnastics and swinging on monkey bars.

One day, Abigail's mom took her to a doctor to see if she had Ehlers-Danlos. Abigail sat nervously, waiting in the exam room. When the doctor came in, he looked at different joints in her body and moved them around. He asked many questions, like "What activities make your body sore?" and "How often do you get hurt?"

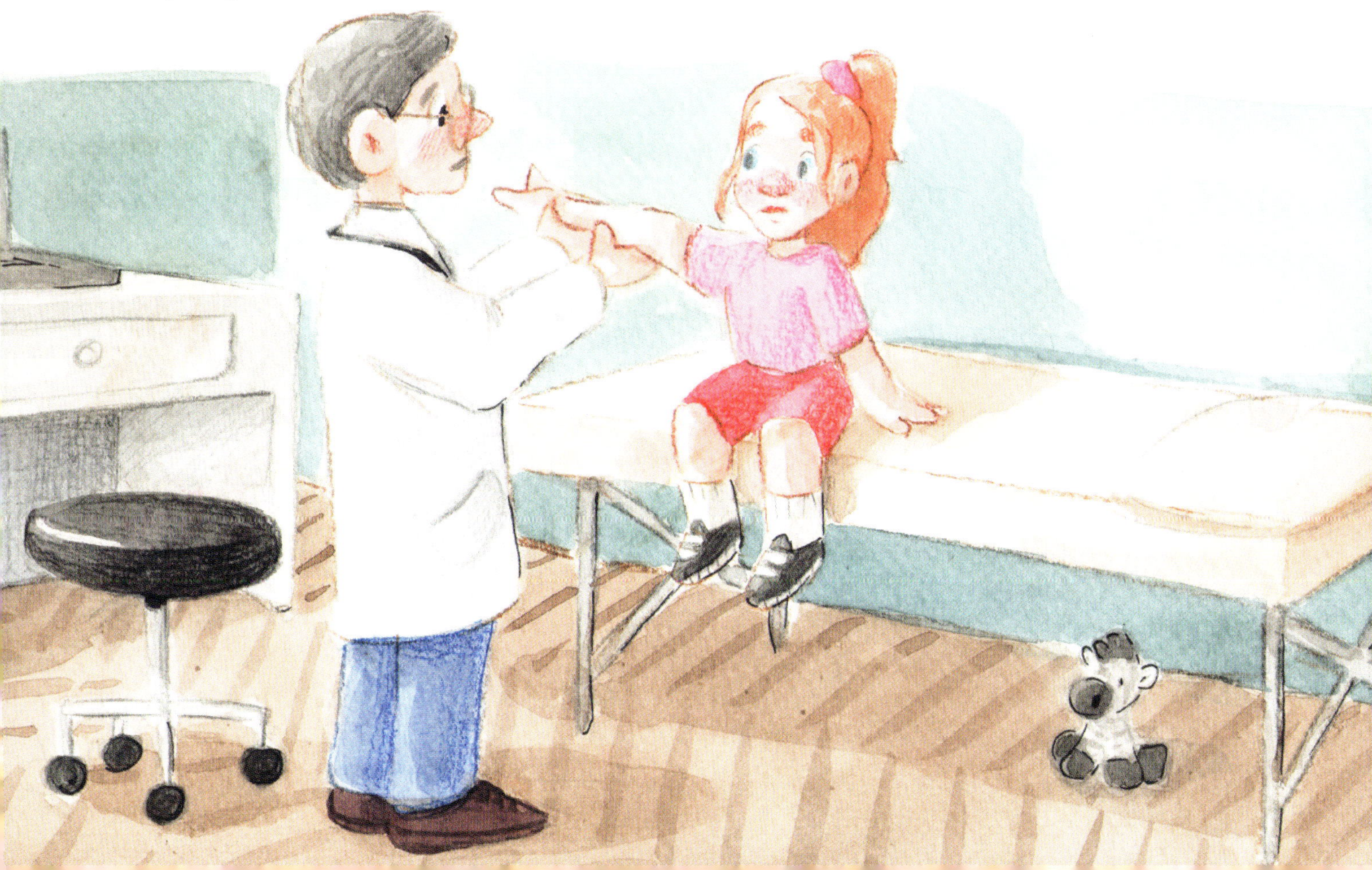

When the exam was over, the doctor said he had some news. He revealed that Abigail had Ehlers-Danlos, just like her mom.

"Abigail, everyone's body produces a special protein called collagen," the doctor explained. "It's like the glue that helps keep our body together and makes our skin, muscles, and organs healthy. But for people who have Ehlers-Danlos, their bodies don't make collagen the way they should, so it can cause stretchy skin and loose joints."

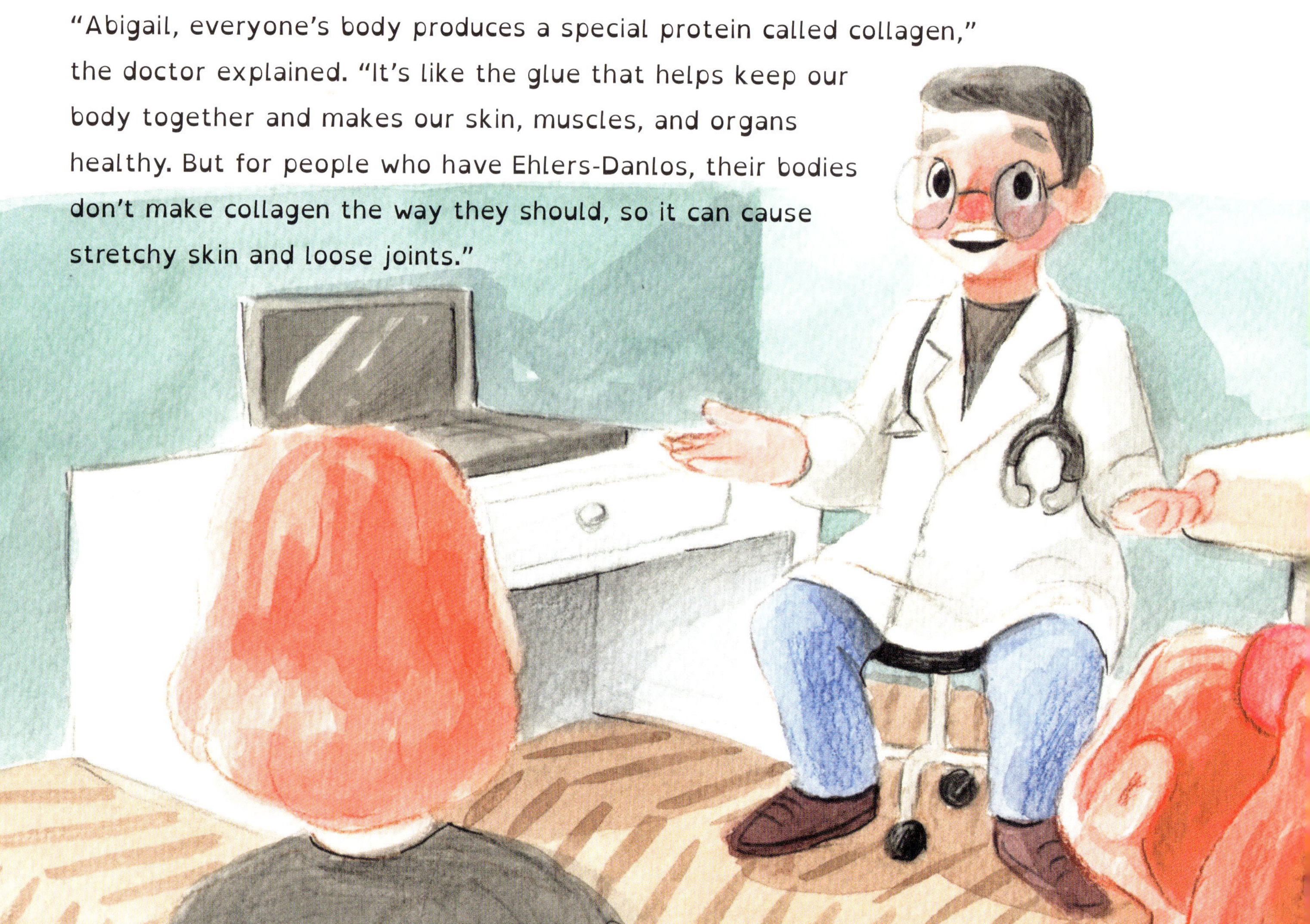

Abigail's mom pointed at her knees and said, "That's why I wear big braces to protect my joints. I also have metal in my feet to keep them strong, so they don't bend too far."

She hugged Abigail. "It's going to be okay."

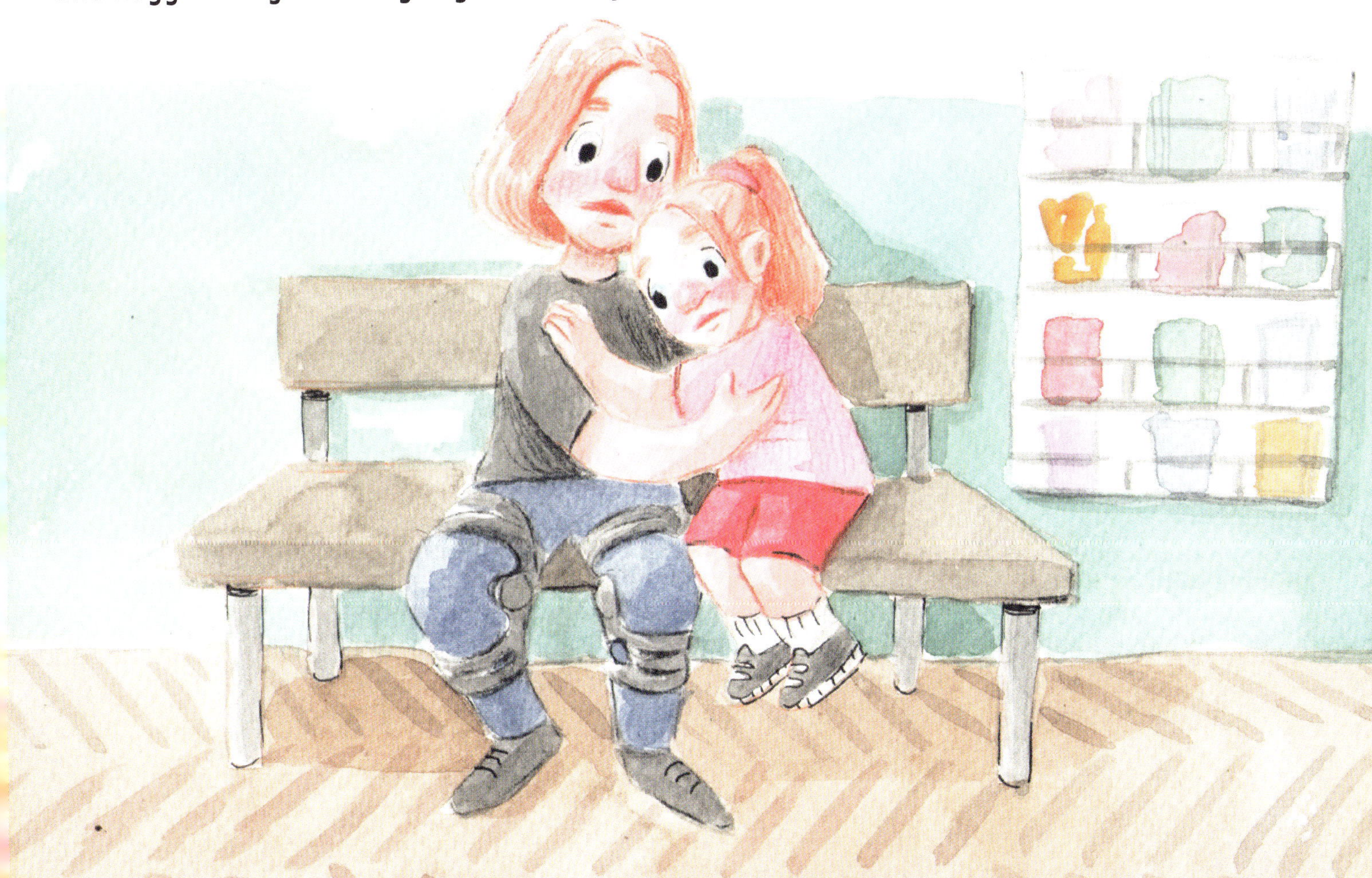

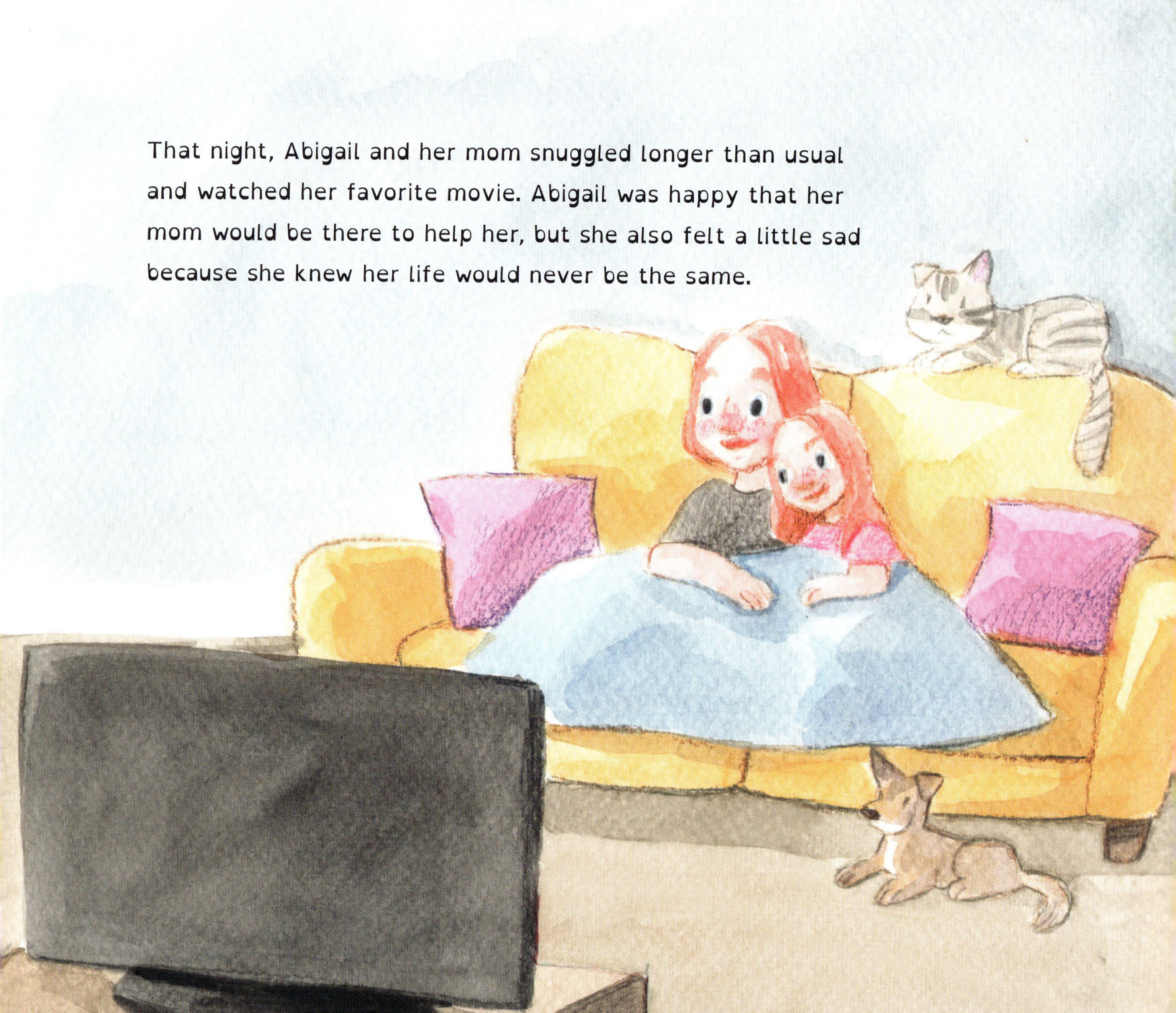

That night, Abigail and her mom snuggled longer than usual and watched her favorite movie. Abigail was happy that her mom would be there to help her, but she also felt a little sad because she knew her life would never be the same.

Soon after, Abigail started using aids in class to help her, like a special chair to sit on and writing tools like a keyboard. She also needed to take walk breaks to help keep her joints from becoming stiff.

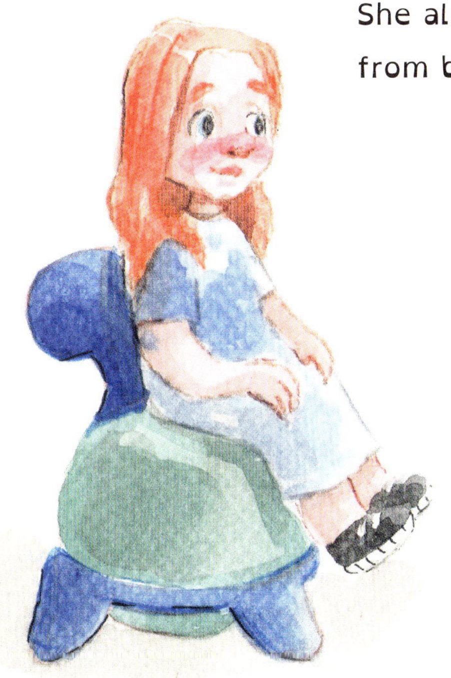

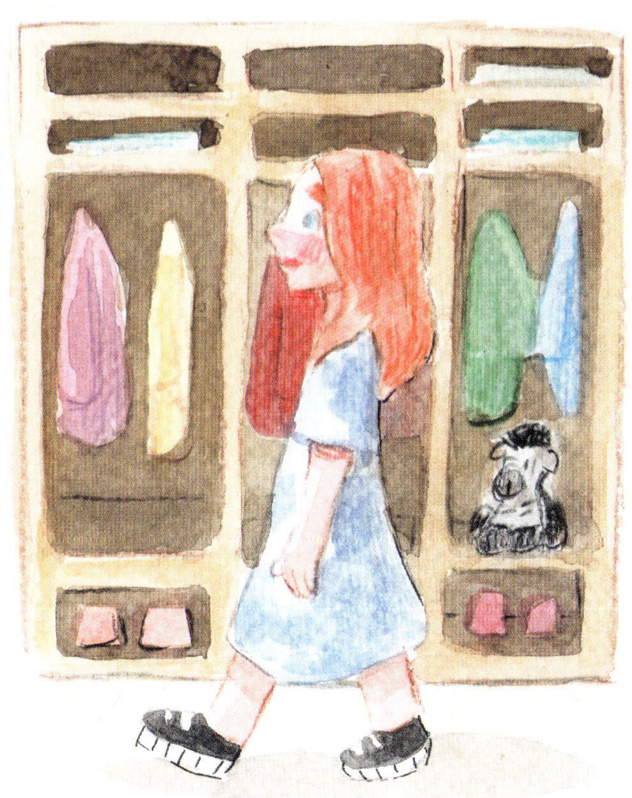

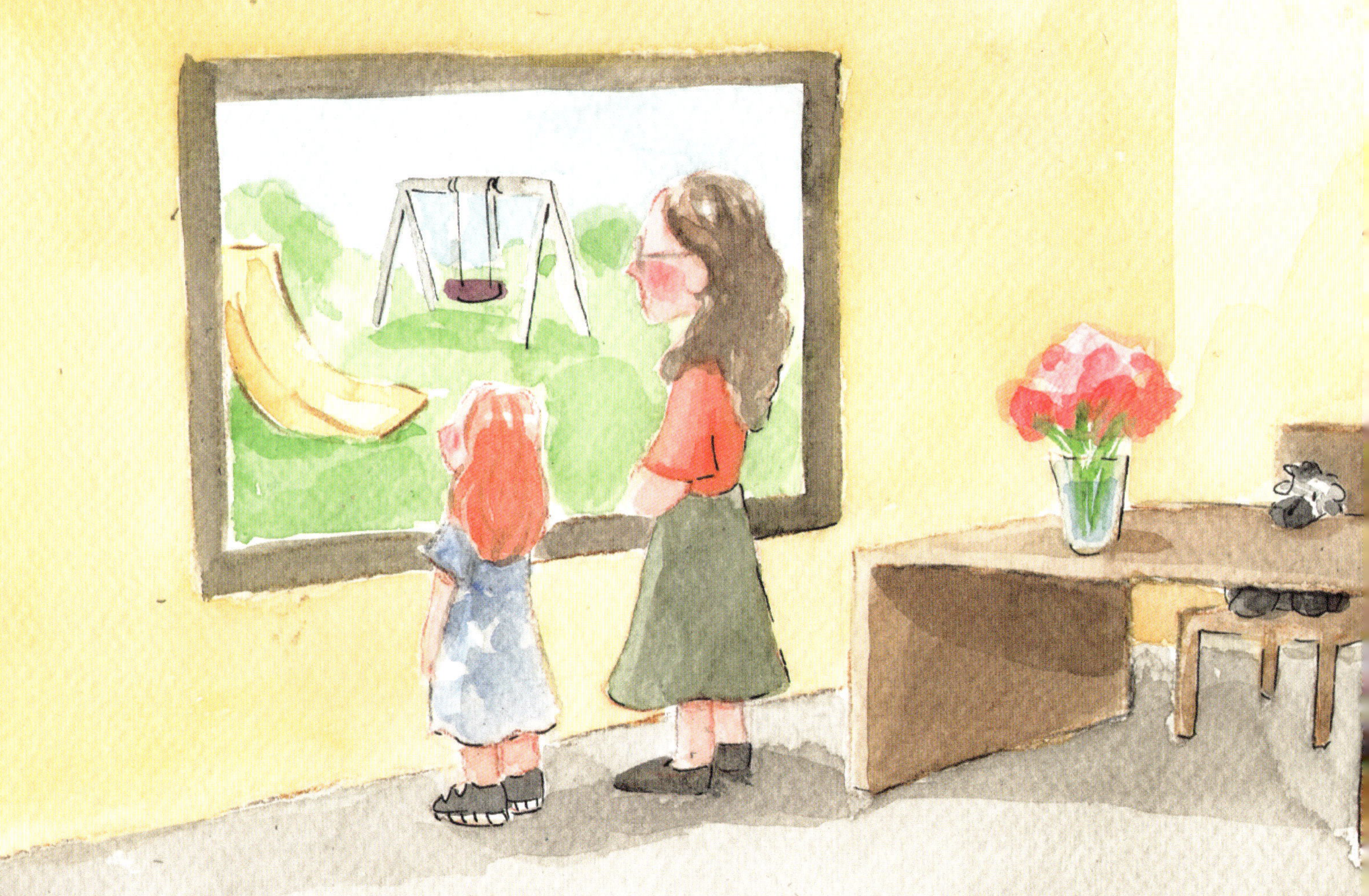

“We will work together to manage it,” her teacher reassured her. “There are lots of fun things you’ll still be able to do. If you are careful, you can play tag, swim, and even play soccer.”

Abigail continued school life as usual, but often felt like her classmates didn't understand. They asked Abigail lots of questions, and she struggled to answer them.

Why do you get to leave class?
Why do you sit on a weird chair?

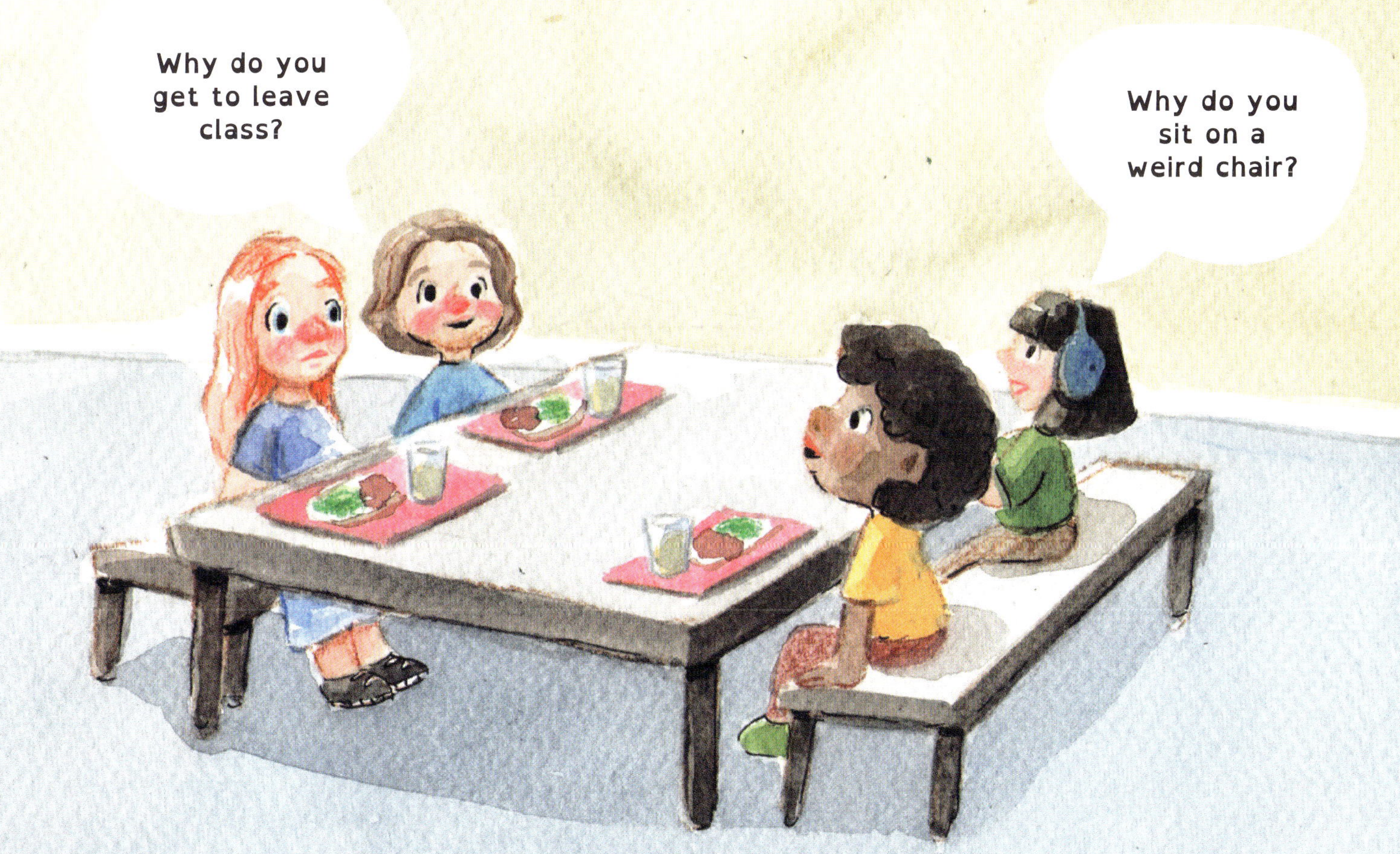

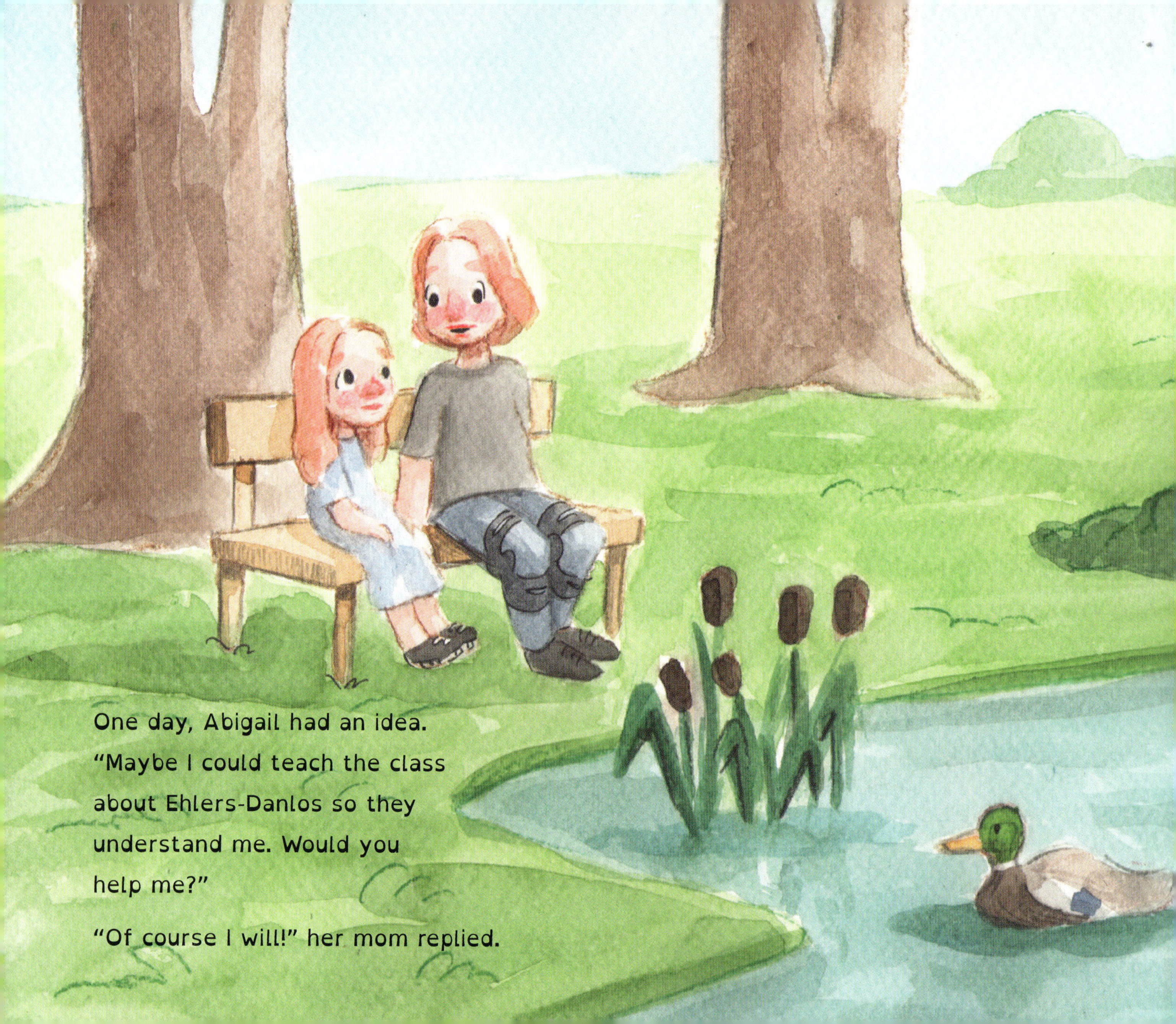

One day, Abigail had an idea. "Maybe I could teach the class about Ehlers-Danlos so they understand me. Would you help me?"

"Of course I will!" her mom replied.

"It can be hard for other people to understand me, too, because I don't look like I have a disability." Her mom smiled warmly. "That's why I talk with everyone to help spread awareness about EDS and invisible disabilities. With a little patience, everyone can understand Ehlers-Danlos."

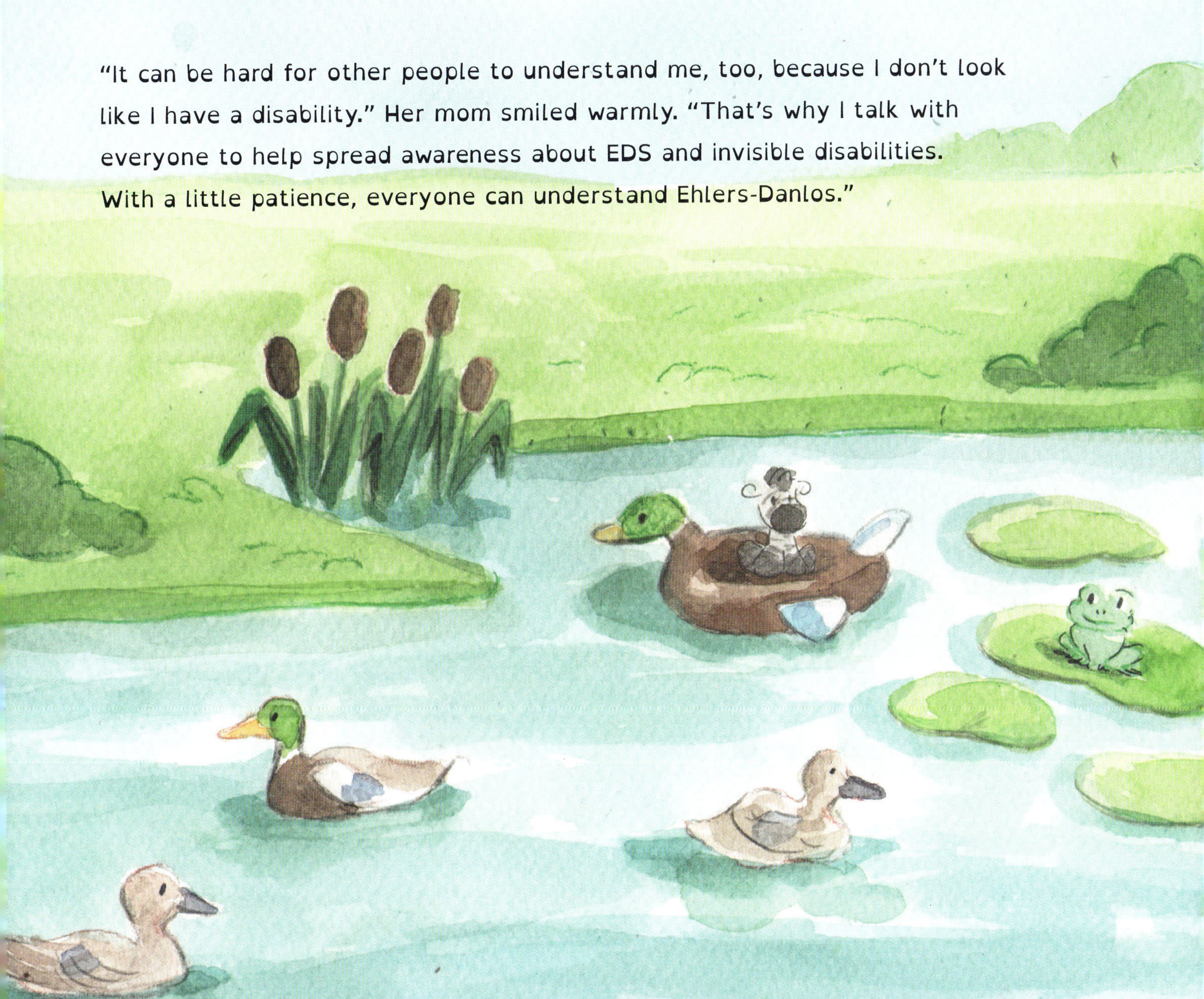

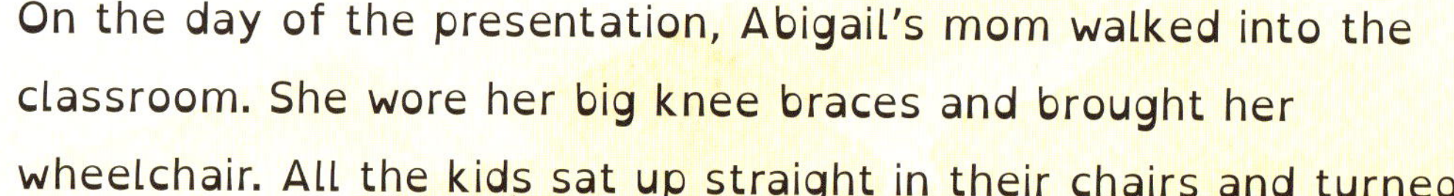

On the day of the presentation, Abigail's mom walked into the classroom. She wore her big knee braces and brought her wheelchair. All the kids sat up straight in their chairs and turned their eyes toward her, curious about why she was there.

Abigail's teacher stood up from her desk and said, "Class, today we have a special guest. Abigail, would you like to tell everyone who our guest is?"

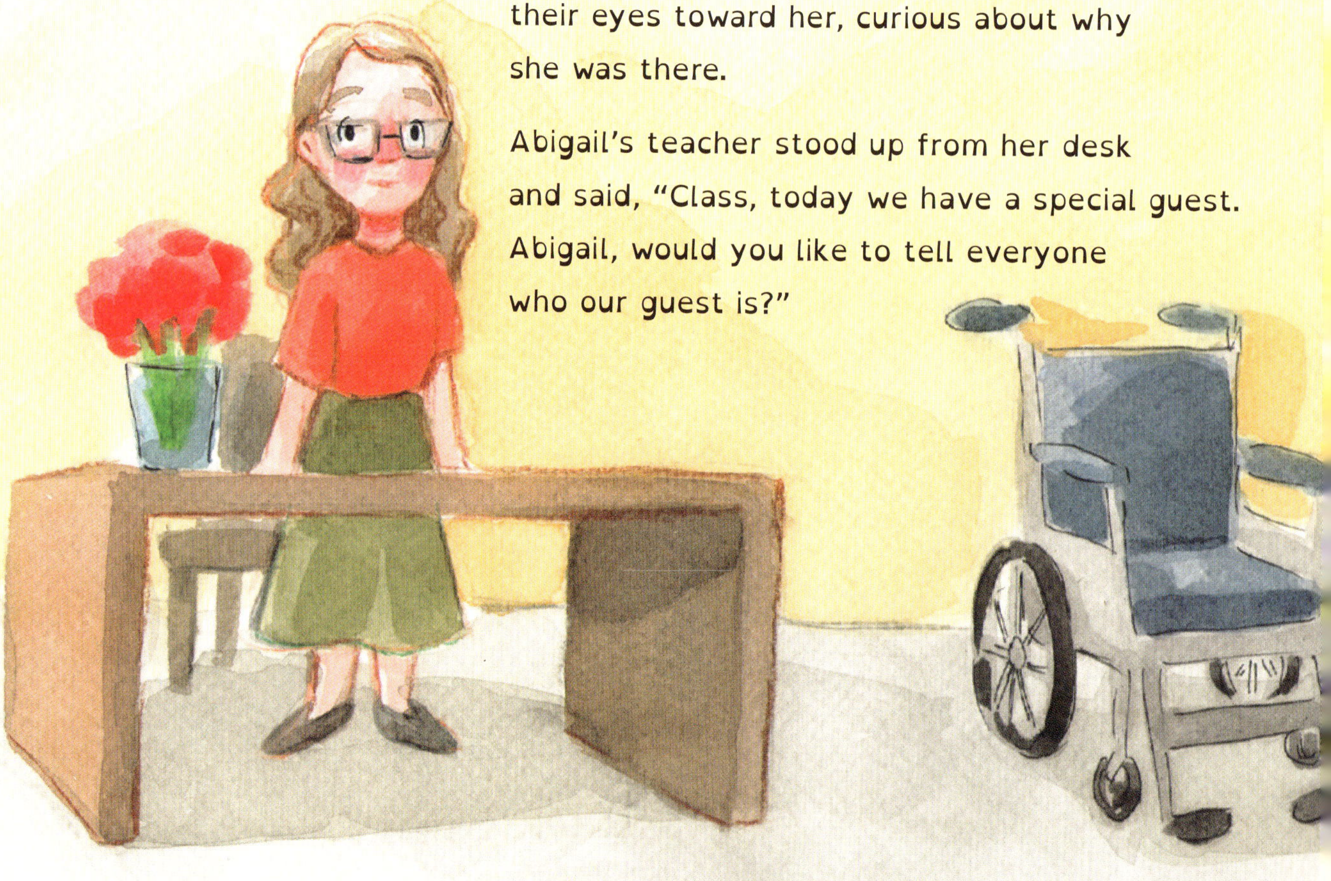

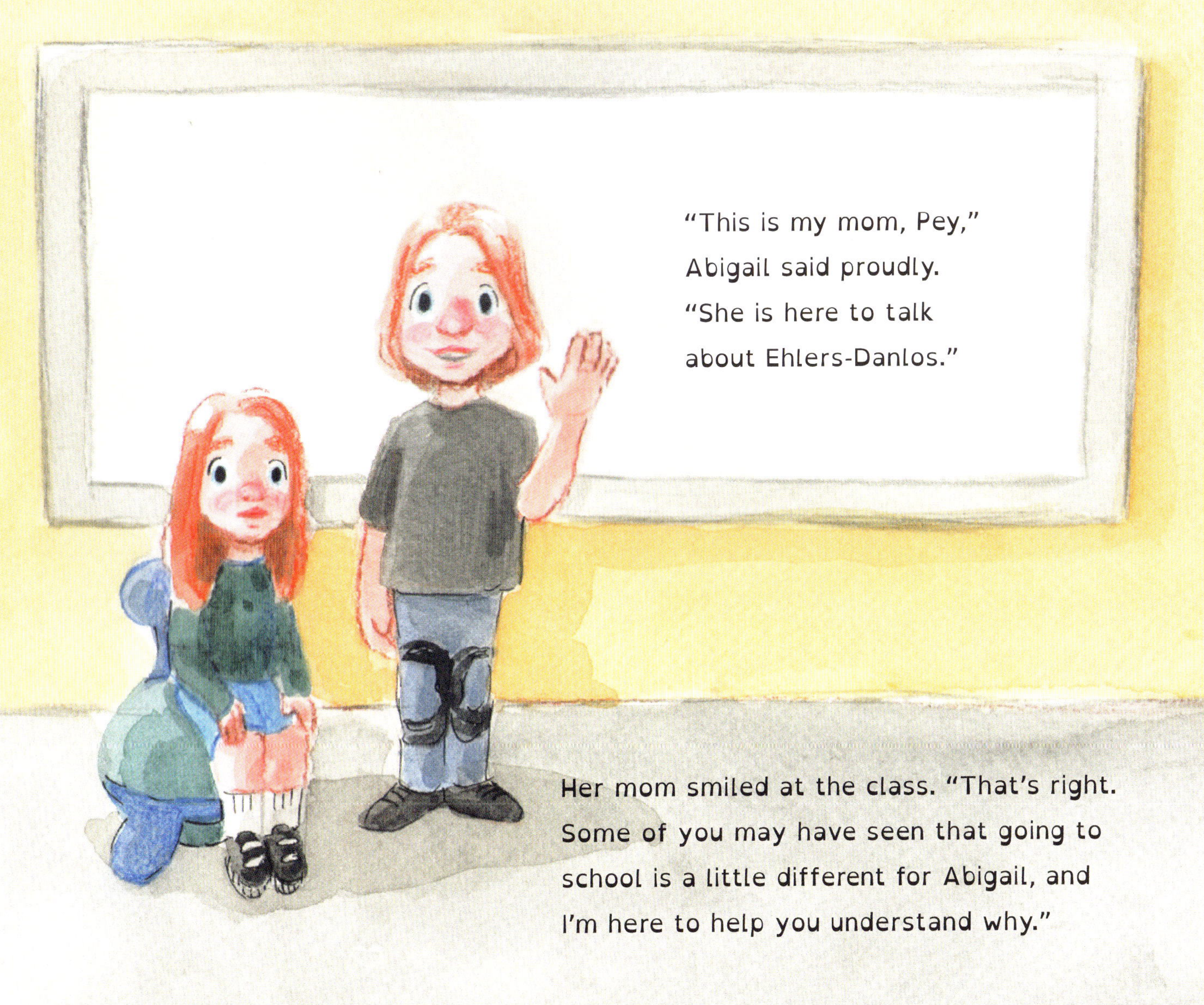

“This is my mom, Pey,” Abigail said proudly. “She is here to talk about Ehlers-Danlos.”

Her mom smiled at the class. “That’s right. Some of you may have seen that going to school is a little different for Abigail, and I’m here to help you understand why.”

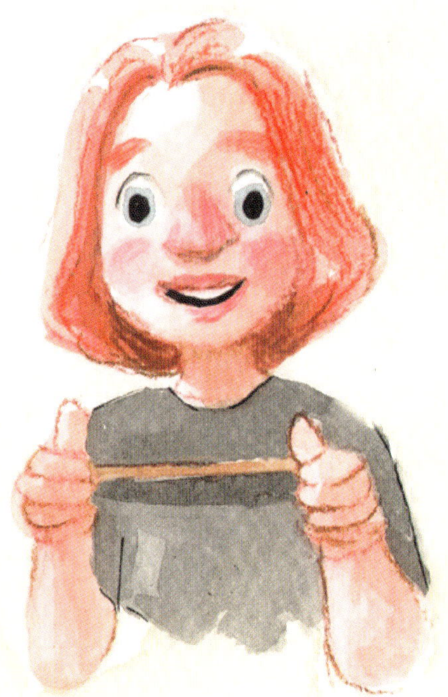

Pey explained to the class about collagen and how people with EDS have bendy bones and stretchy skin.

"Let's take a rubber band as an example. With typical people, their rubber band stretches within a normal range. Then, over time, when it is much older, it may snap. For people with EDS, the rubber band is too stretchy. What do you think happens to it?" she asked the class.

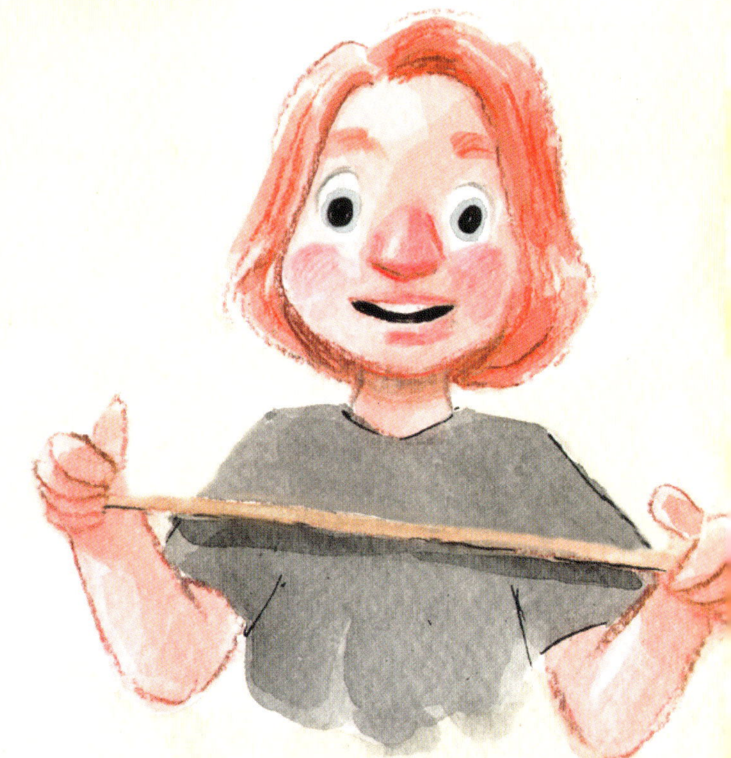

“It won’t be strong,” a boy said.

“It’d break easily!” another student exclaimed.

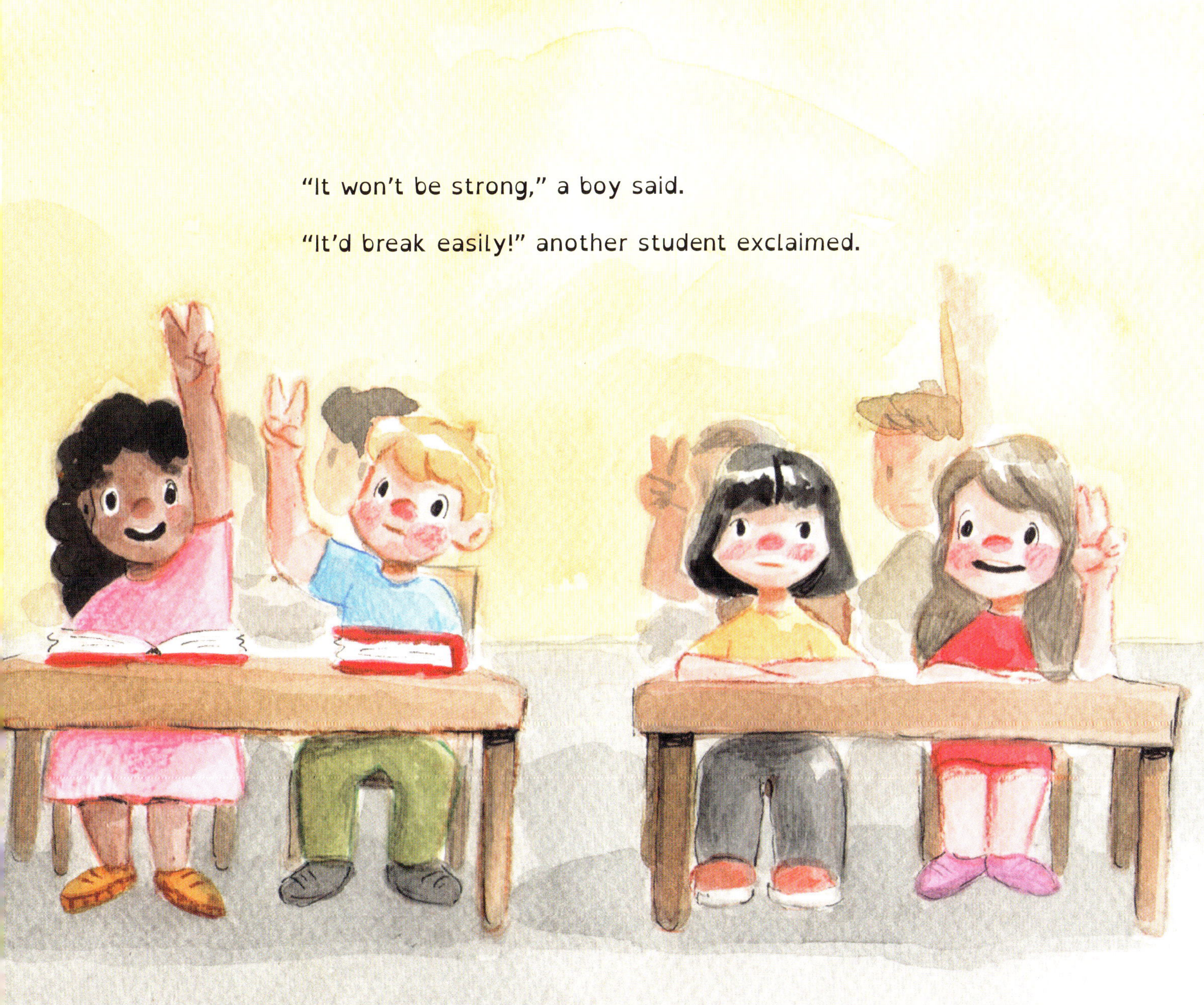

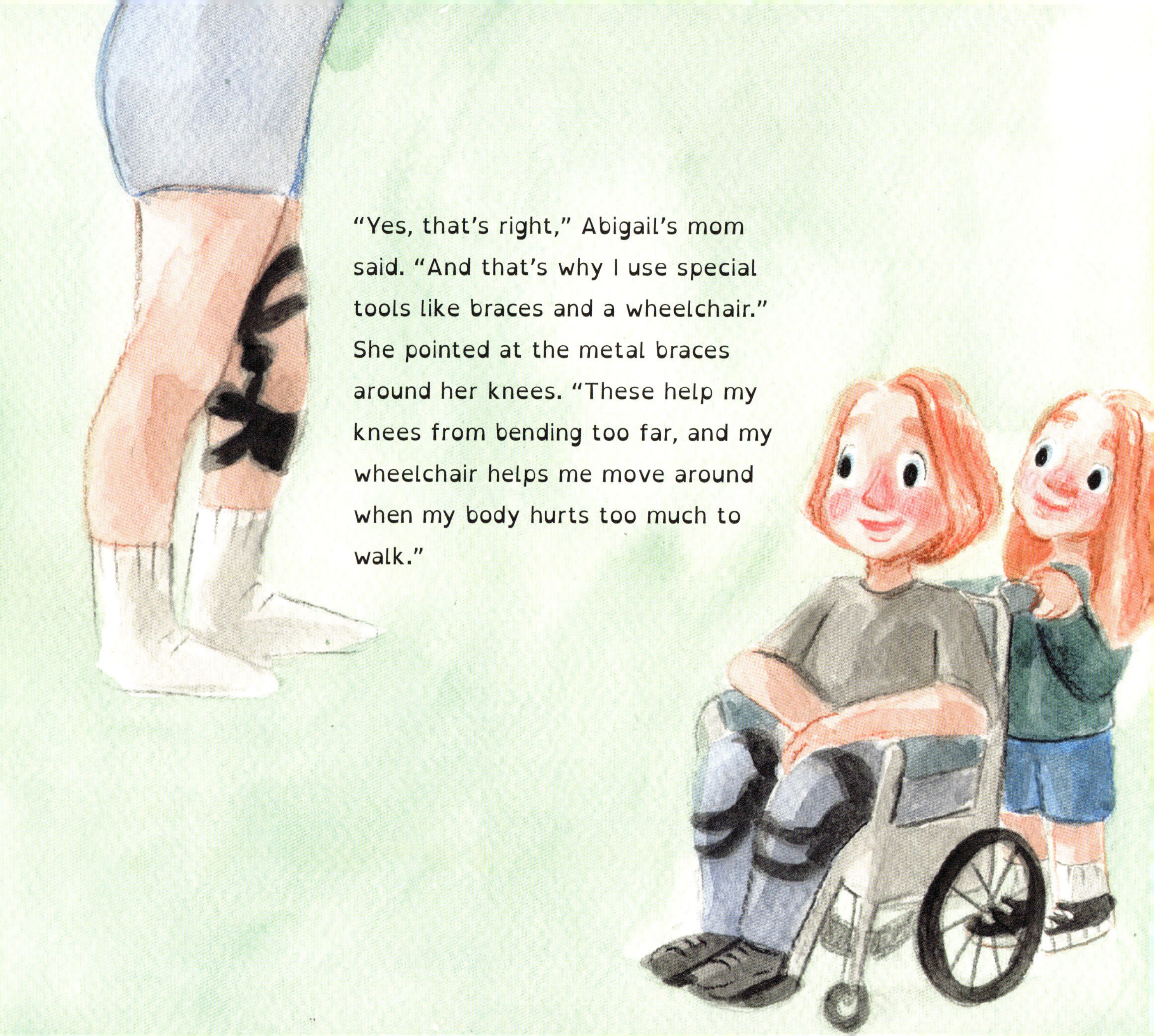

"Yes, that's right," Abigail's mom said. "And that's why I use special tools like braces and a wheelchair." She pointed at the metal braces around her knees. "These help my knees from bending too far, and my wheelchair helps me move around when my body hurts too much to walk."

“EDS isn’t a reason for Abigail to feel sad or isolated,” she continued. “She has a lot of tools to help keep her safe and prevent injuries.”

“When my wrists ache from writing a lot, I can use a keyboard,” Abigail added.

“Is that why our teacher sometimes helps you write?” a girl asked.

Abigail nodded. “I get a lot of support from school to help me learn the best I can.”

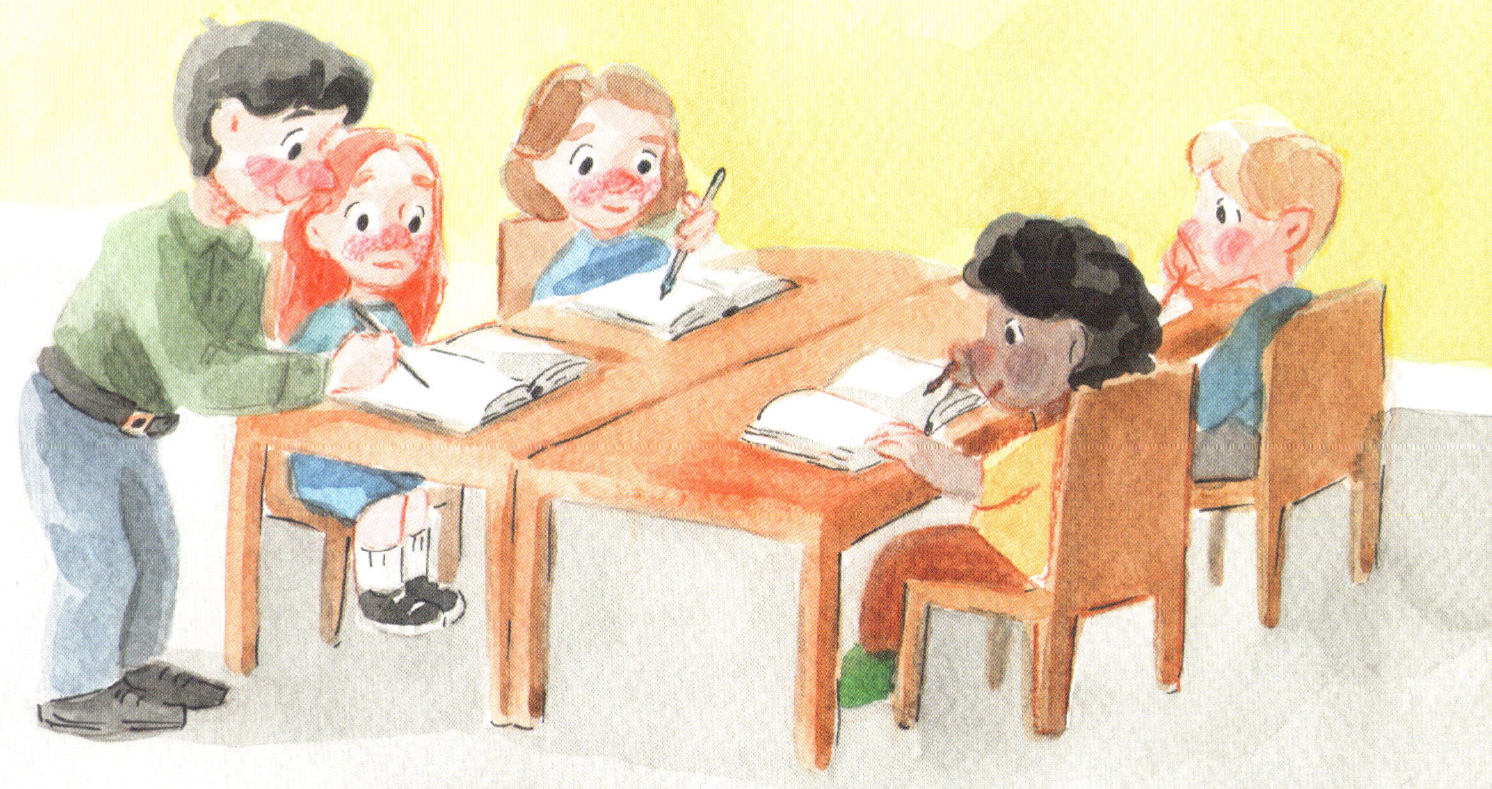

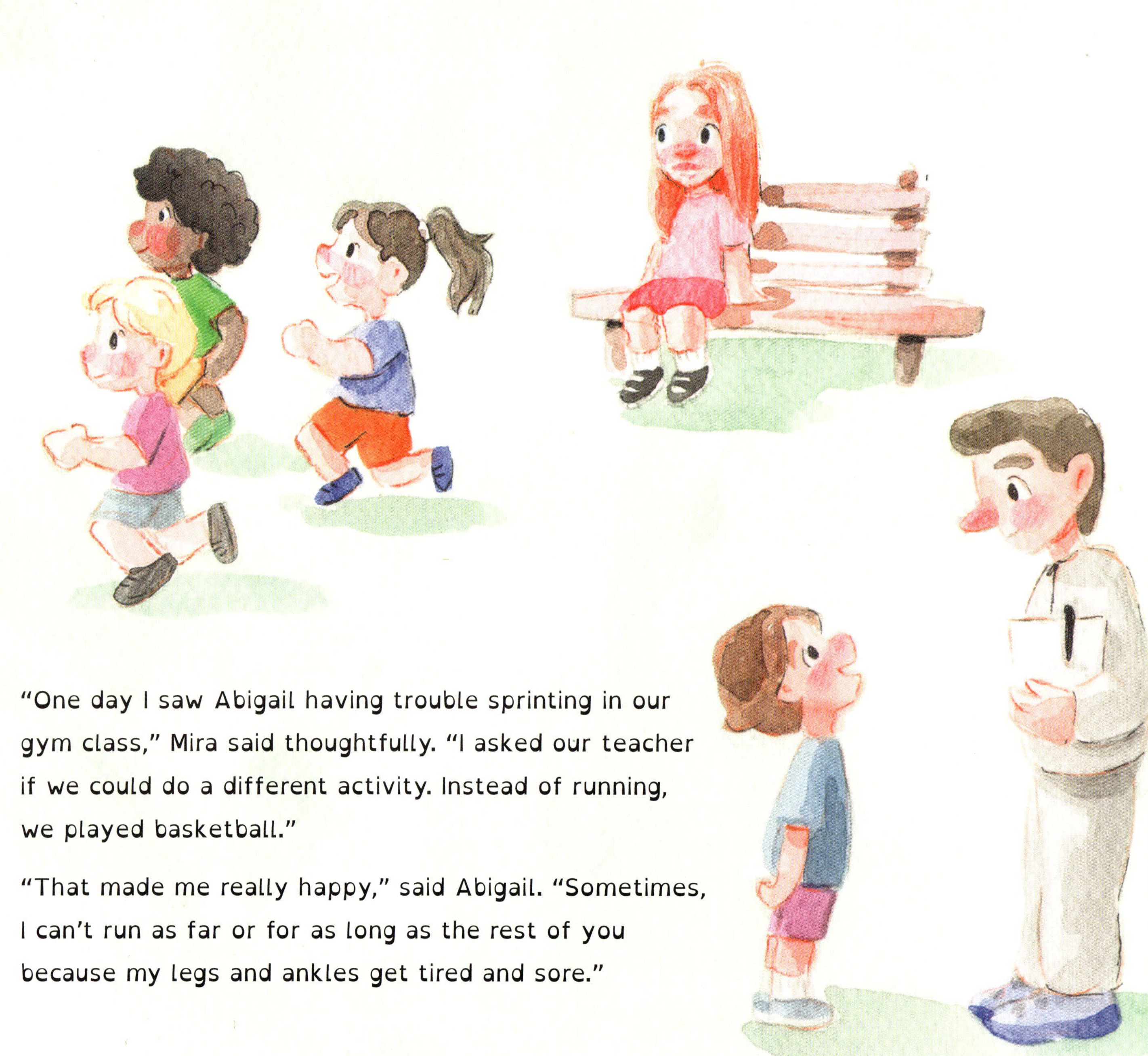

“One day I saw Abigail having trouble sprinting in our gym class,” Mira said thoughtfully. “I asked our teacher if we could do a different activity. Instead of running, we played basketball.”

“That made me really happy,” said Abigail. “Sometimes, I can’t run as far or for as long as the rest of you because my legs and ankles get tired and sore.”

"I have many other people to help me," said Abigail.

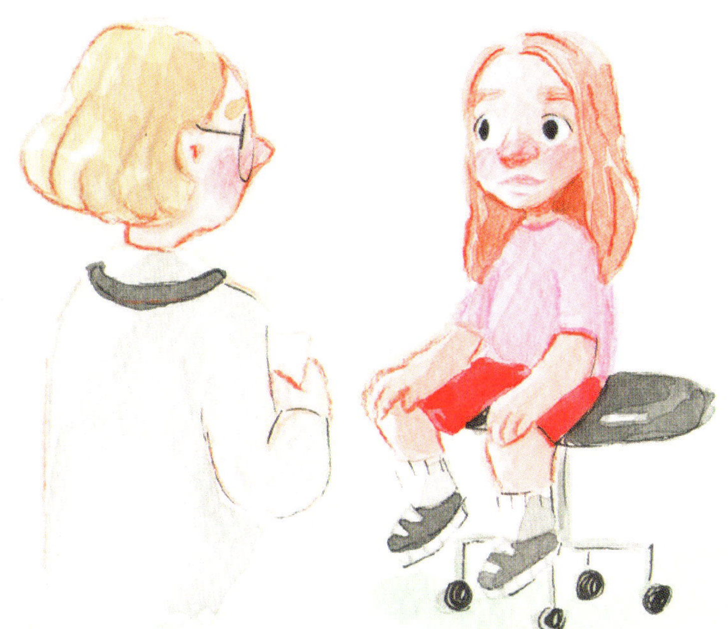

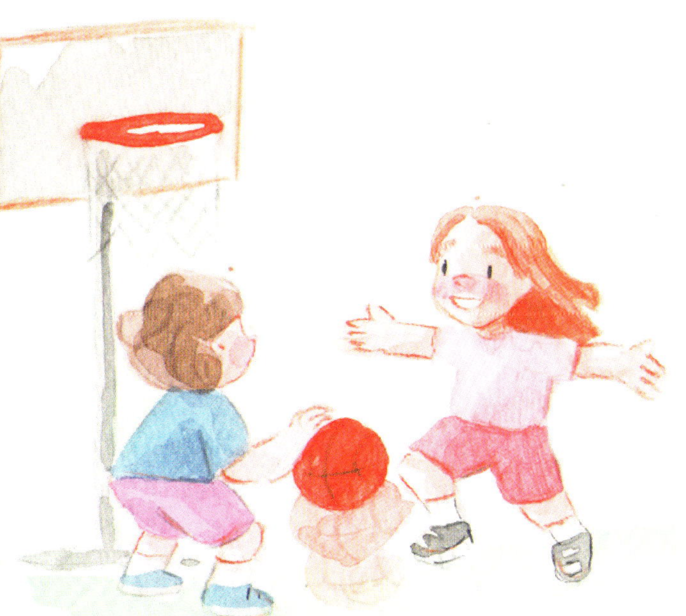

"The physical therapist helps make my muscles strong through different exercises. When I fall or hurt myself, the nurse makes sure that little injuries don't turn into big ones."

"Abigail also has speech therapy," her mom added. "People with Ehlers-Danlos can get infections easily because our skin is fragile and takes a while to heal. When Abigail was a baby, she had many ear infections, making it difficult to learn certain sounds. Imagine being underwater in a pool and trying to hear someone speaking from above the water."

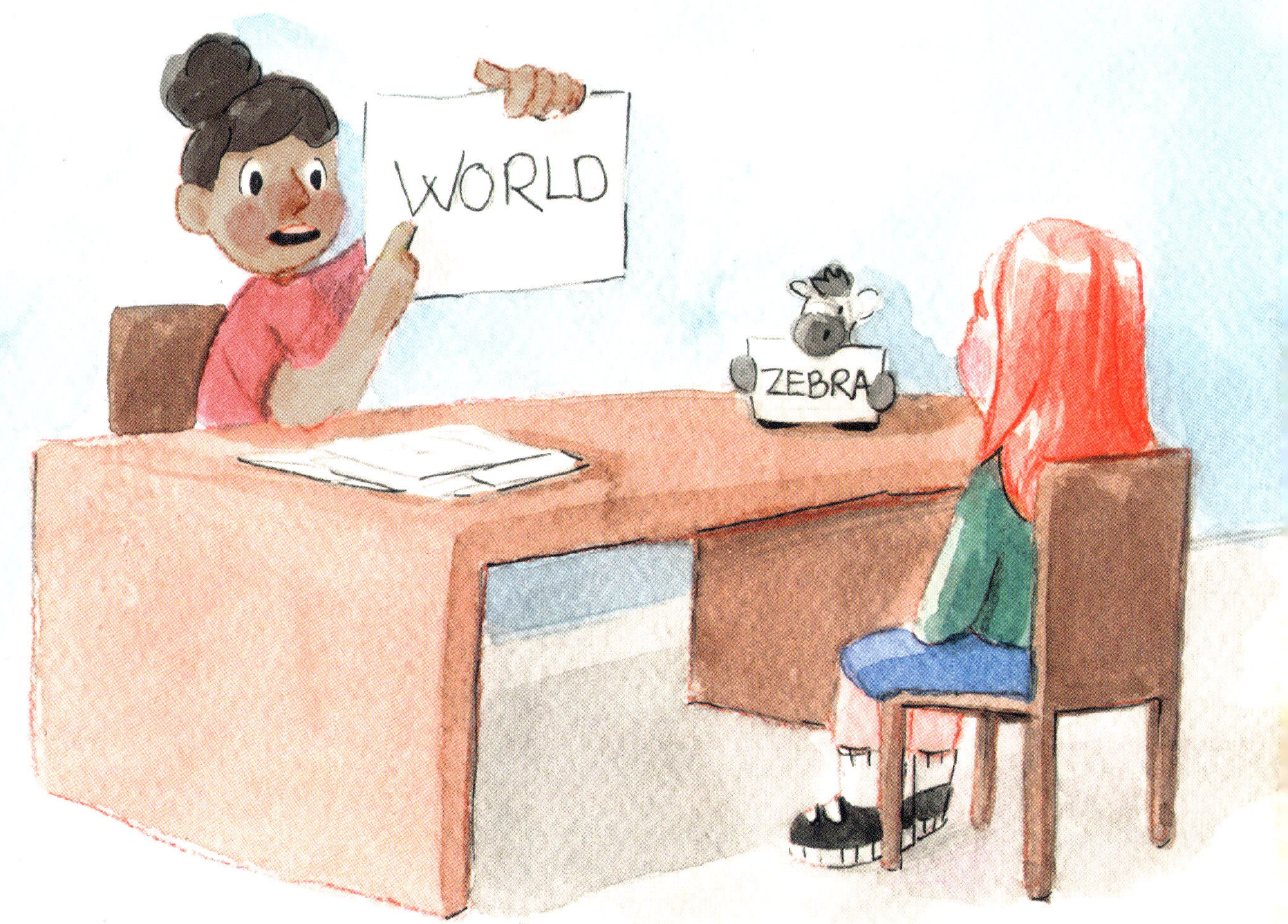

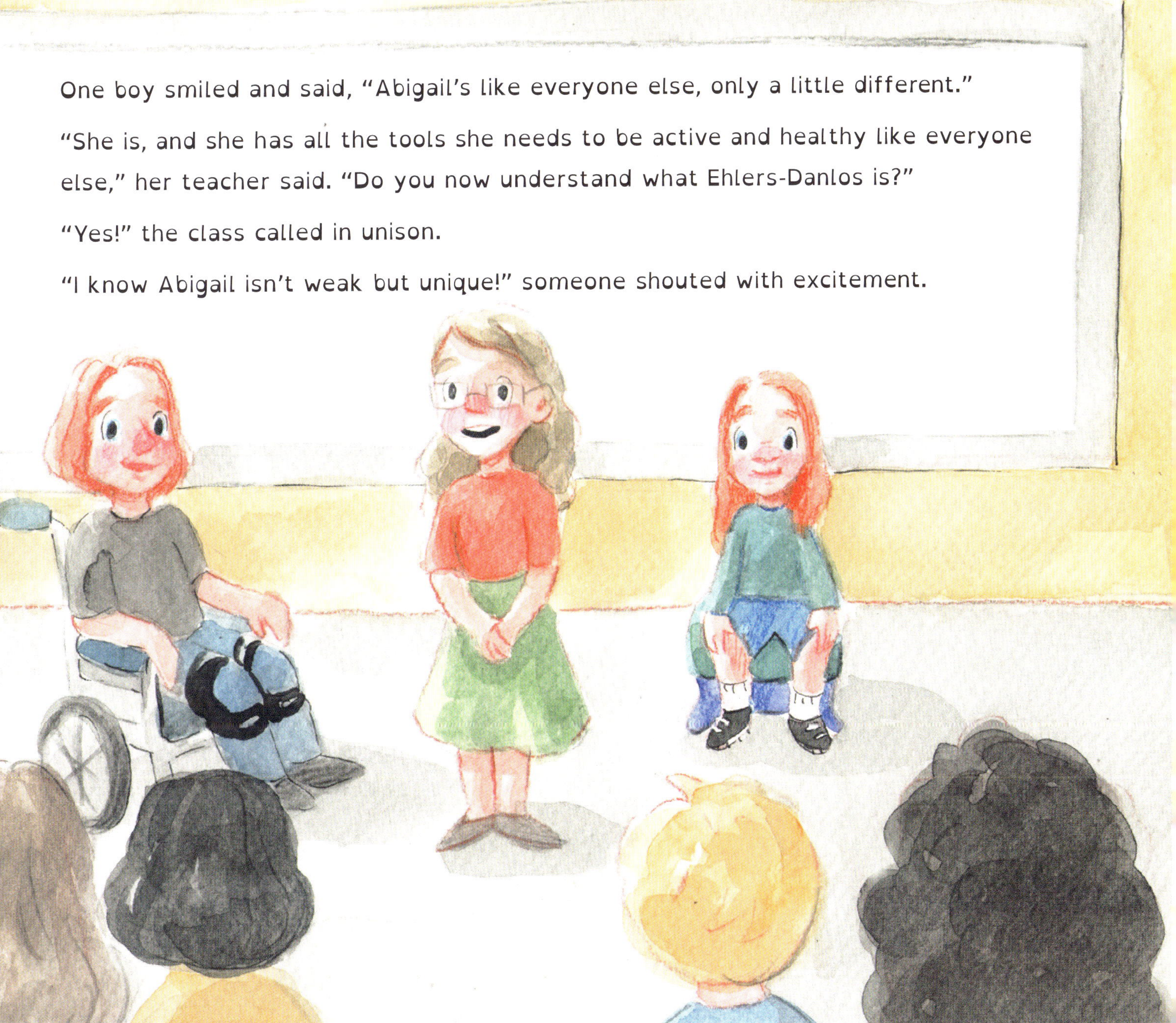

One boy smiled and said, “Abigail’s like everyone else, only a little different.”

“She is, and she has all the tools she needs to be active and healthy like everyone else,” her teacher said. “Do you now understand what Ehlers-Danlos is?”

“Yes!” the class called in unison.

“I know Abigail isn’t weak but unique!” someone shouted with excitement.

As Abigail walked her mom out of the classroom, she gazed at her mom with admiration.

"I love you," she mouthed to her mom with her brightest smile.

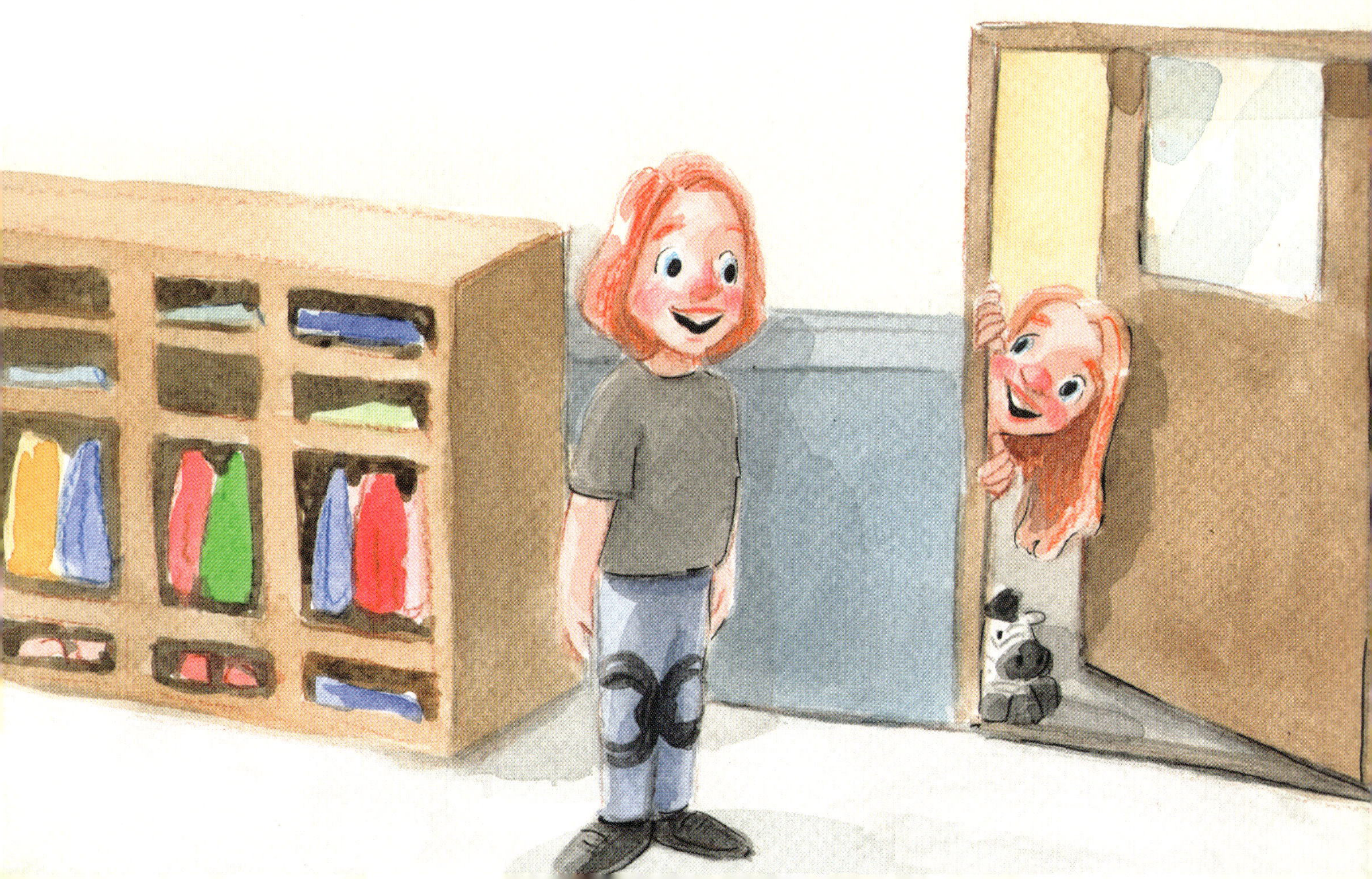

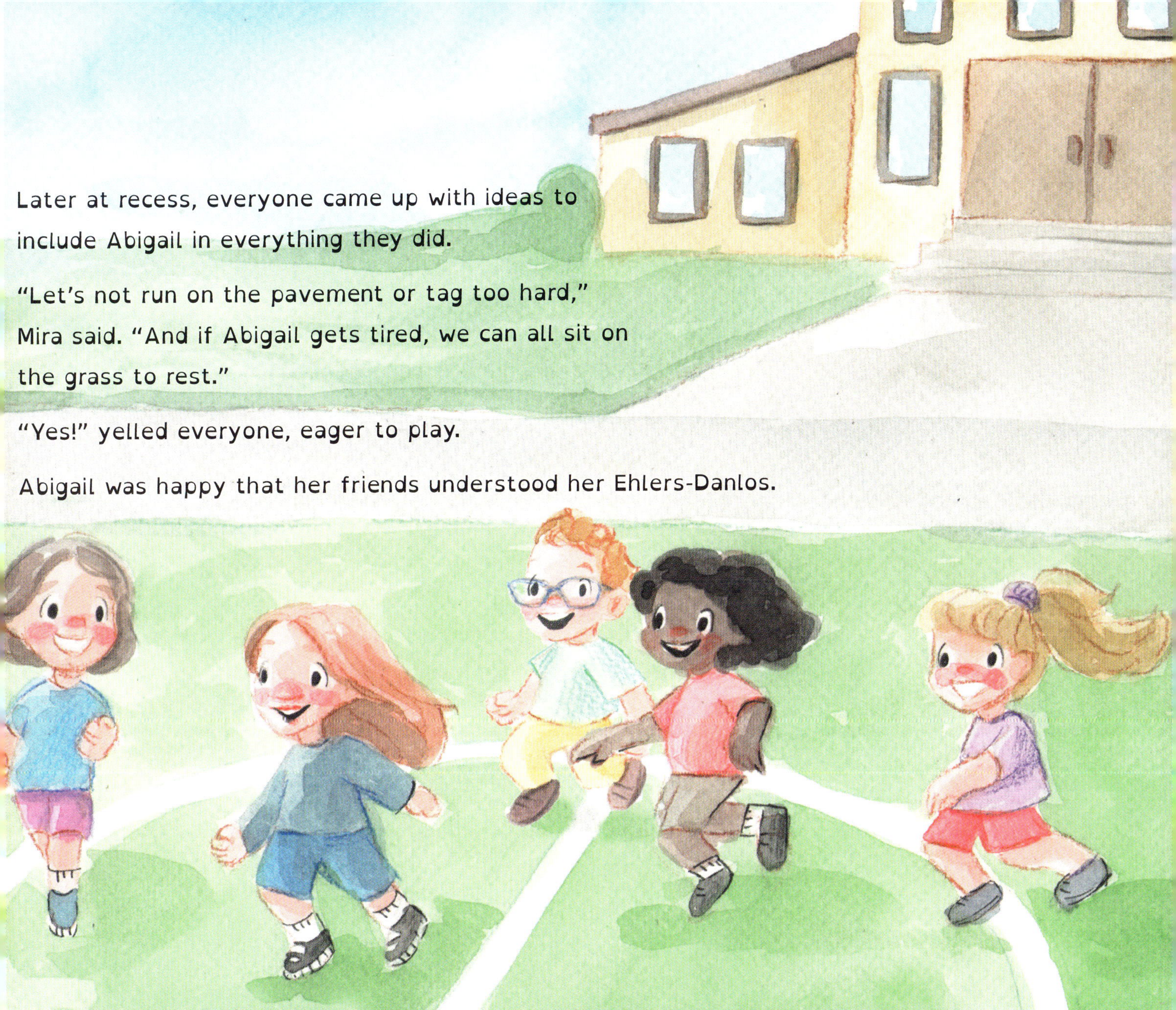

Later at recess, everyone came up with ideas to include Abigail in everything they did.

"Let's not run on the pavement or tag too hard," Mira said. "And if Abigail gets tired, we can all sit on the grass to rest."

"Yes!" yelled everyone, eager to play.

Abigail was happy that her friends understood her Ehlers-Danlos.

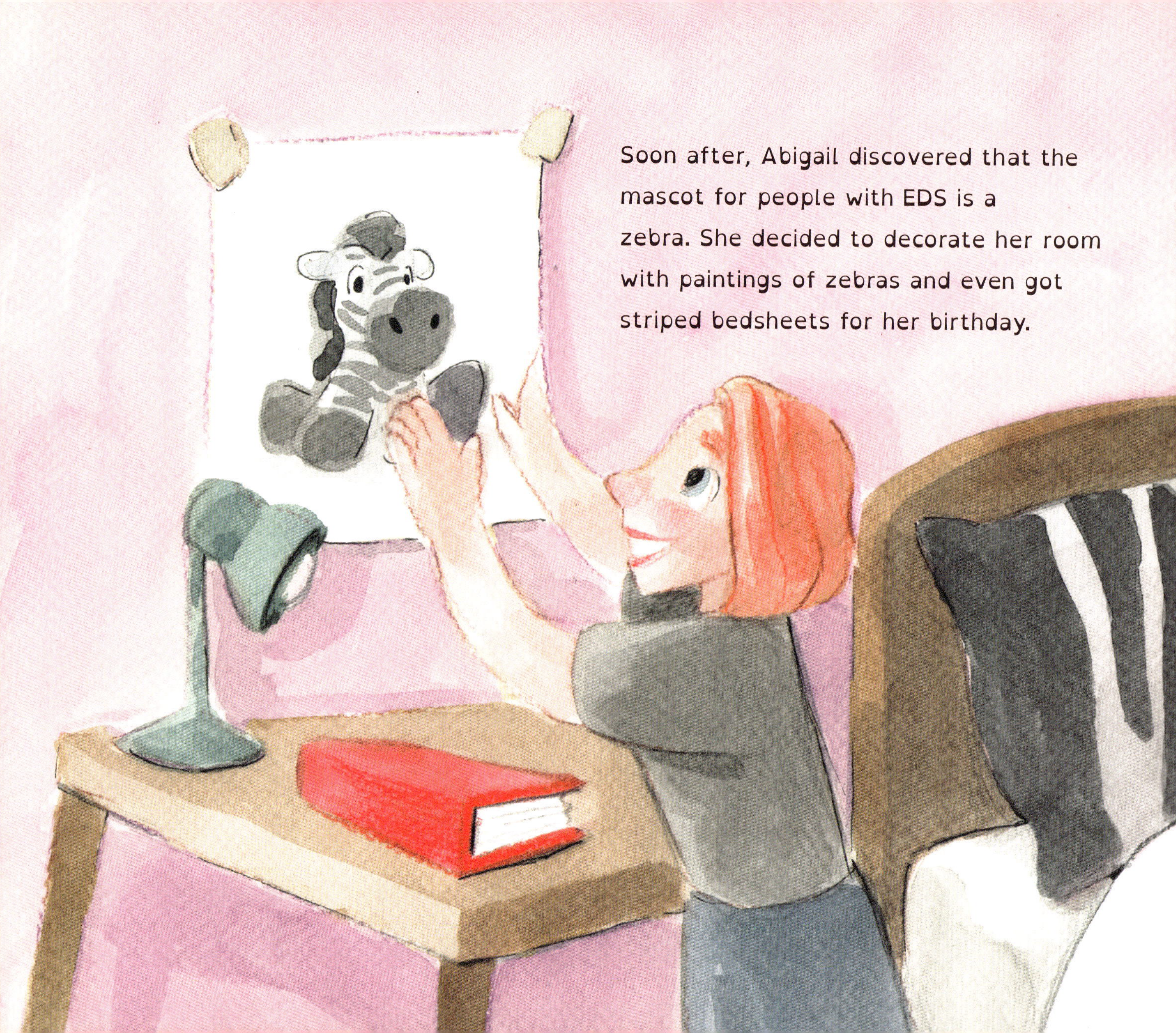

Soon after, Abigail discovered that the mascot for people with EDS is a zebra. She decided to decorate her room with paintings of zebras and even got striped bedsheets for her birthday.

Abigail received a stuffed zebra she named “Spirit” from Sofia’s Helping Hand, a charity started by a girl who also has Ehlers-Danlos.

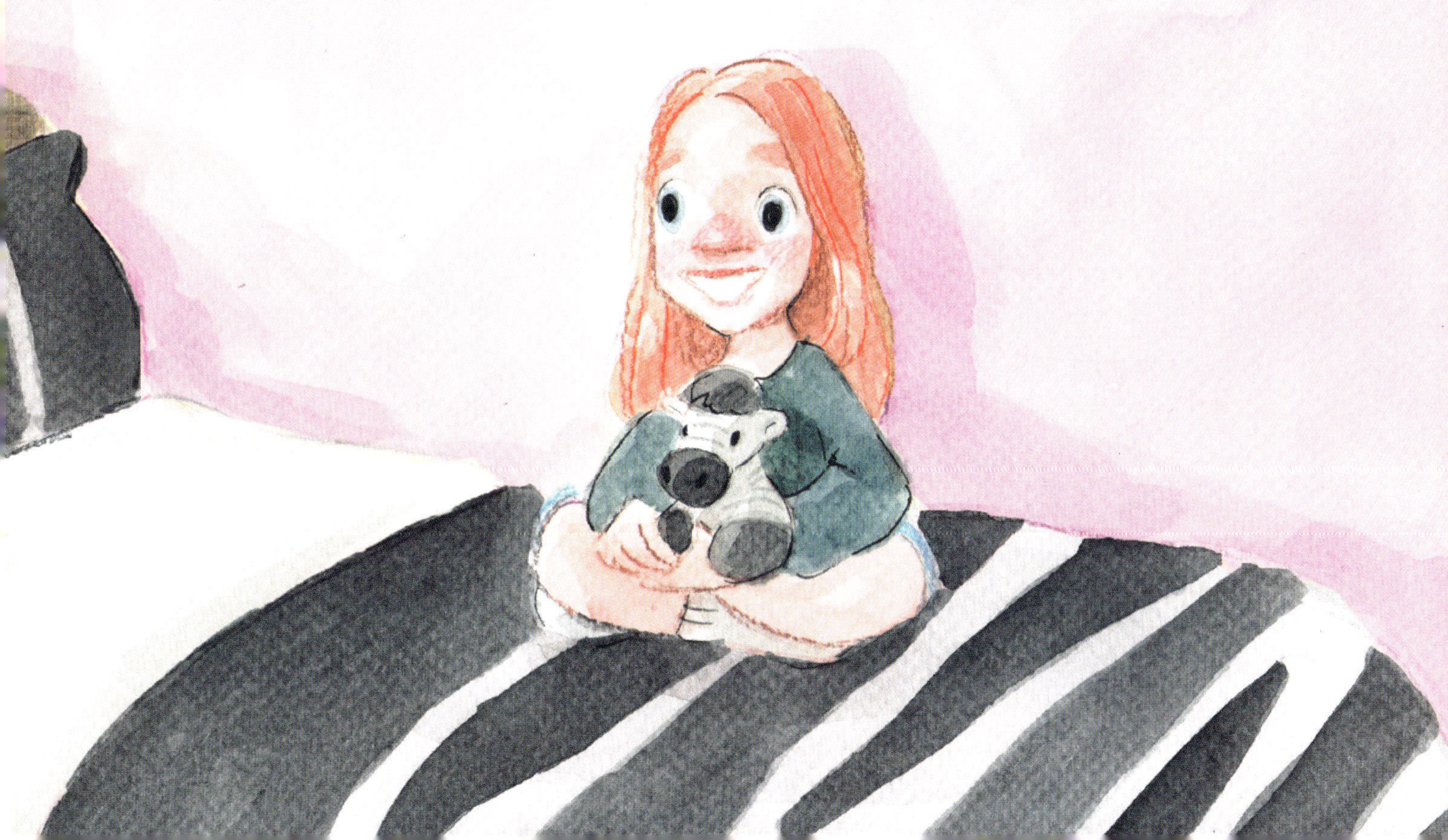

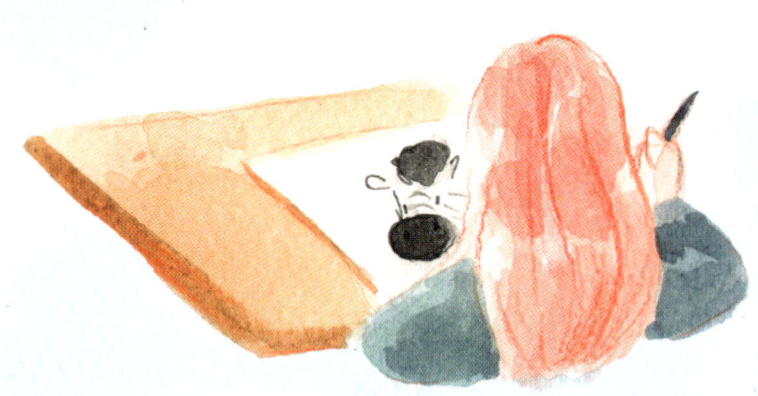

Abigail's mom found a pen pal group for kids with chronic illnesses, and soon Abigail had friends from all over the world who also have Ehlers-Danlos. They formed a tight bond, calling themselves the "Little Zebras," writing letters and sending drawings to each other.

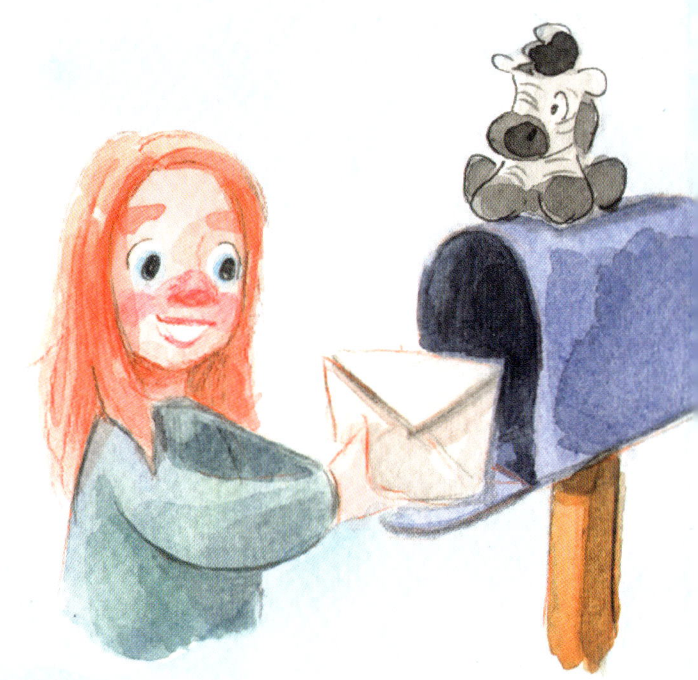

Although there are days Abigail feels frustrated and sad, she knows she isn't alone. She has her mom, friends, and the "Little Zebras" to support her.

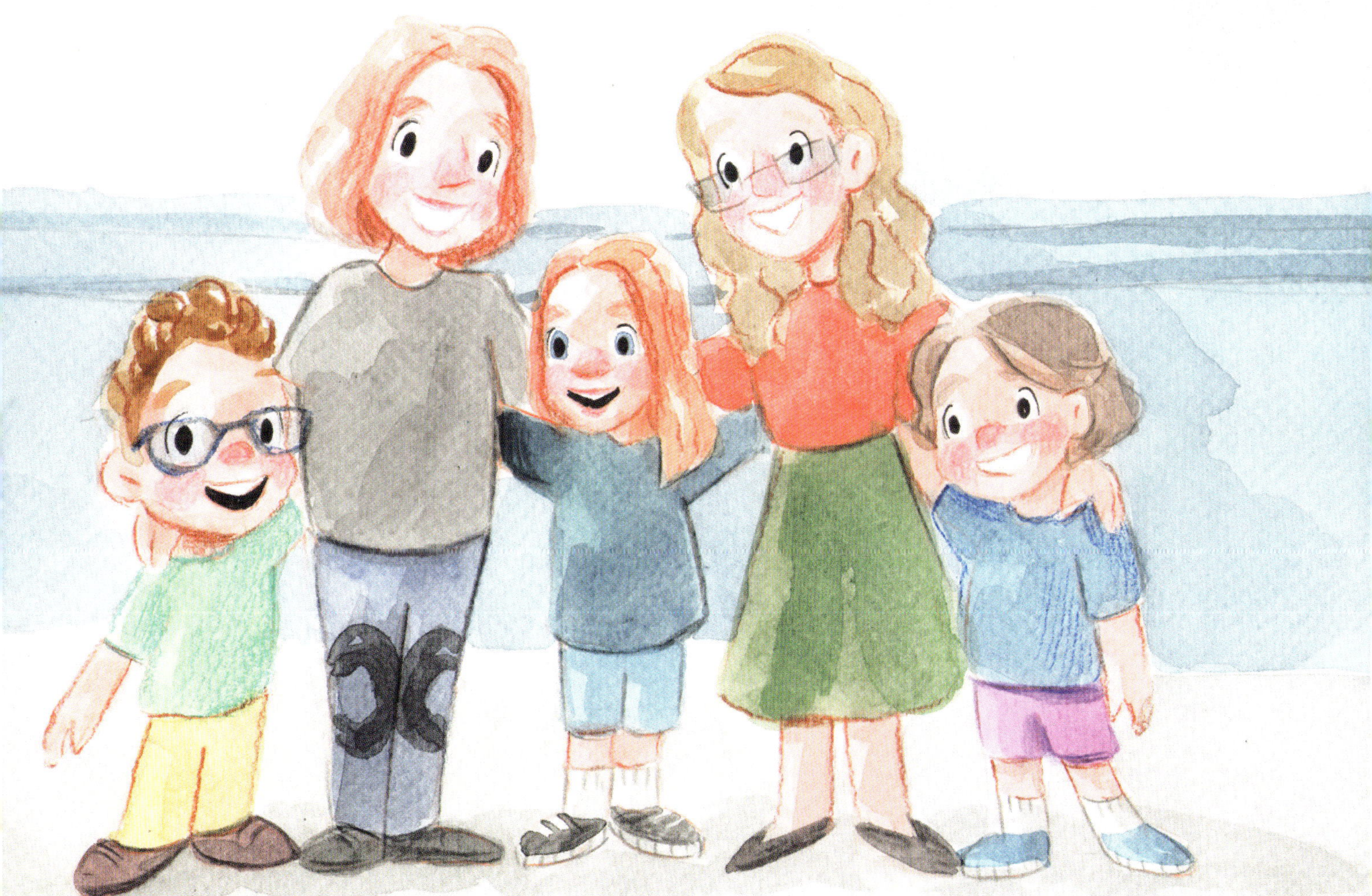

About Ehlers-Danlos Syndrome

(Pronounced like eh·lrz dan·lowz syndrome)

Ehlers-Danlos Syndrome, or EDS, is a group of thirteen tissue-connectivity disorders that affect the body's collagen, which makes skin, tissue, and muscles healthy. While EDS seems rare, many organizations believe it's more common than we think.

Every type of Ehlers-Danlos is unique, sometimes with subtle symptoms, so it can be hard to diagnose. Pey and Abigail have the most common type, Hypermobile Ehlers-Danlos, or hEDS.

There are many ways to be a great ally to people with visible and invisible disabilities. Listen to the experiences of people who have chronic illnesses. Many people have invisible disabilities you can't see, so don't judge based on what people look like. If you see someone who appears to be struggling with a task, ask before helping, and be respectful if they say no. If a place seems like it might be hard for wheelchair users and people with disabilities to navigate, ask questions about accessibility–you might help make a change! Most importantly, celebrate diversity. Our differences make us special.

For more information about EDS, visit the Ehlers-Danlos Society's website at **www.ehlers-danlos.com.**

Five percent of all profit from book sales will be donated to the Ehlers-Danlos Society.

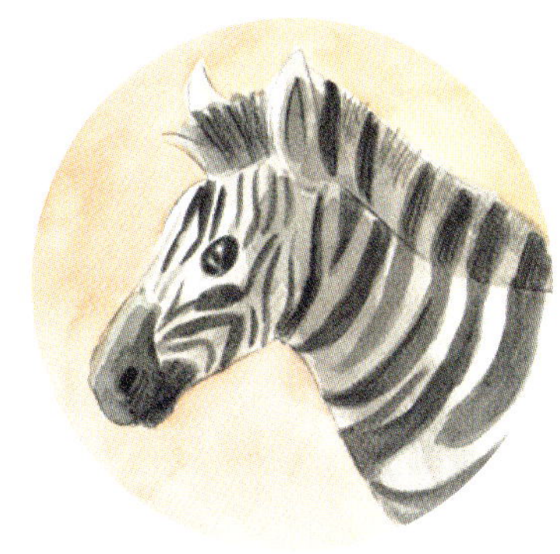

Discussion Questions

łave you ever heard of the term "invisible disabilities"? What do you think it means?

What are some examples of invisible disabilities?

łow do you think an invisible disability might impact someone's daily life?

)o you think people with invisible disabilities are treated differently than those with lisabilities you can see? How do you think it makes them feel?

łow can we be a good friend to someone who has disabilities?

Visit **www.spooniekids.co.uk** *for a great kid-friendly exercise on how disabilities can impact daily living.*

Why Representation Matters

A Note for Adults

Inclusive representation in children's books matters immensely because it shapes young minds, influences self-perception, and fosters empathy and understanding. When children see characters who look like them, come from similar backgrounds, or share their experiences, it validates their identities and instills a sense of belonging, helping to boost their self-esteem and confidence.

When children read about characters with experiences and challenges different from their own, it broadens their horizons and introduces them to diverse cultures, perspectives, and abilities, encouraging them to embrace differences and cultivate an inclusive worldview.

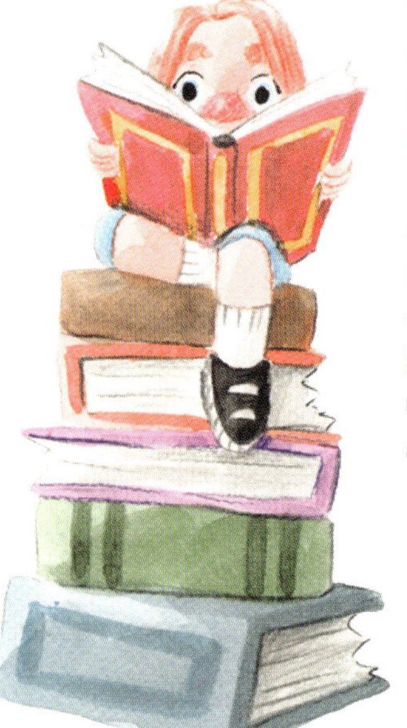

Overall, representation in literature is not just about reflecting the world as it is, but also about shaping it into a more equitable and compassionate place for future generations. It makes all the difference in helping our kids show up for each other, so they can grow up unafraid, undeterred, and utterly confident in their right to be loved and belong.

Acknowledgments

A heartfelt thanks for joining us on this literary journey, helping to plant seeds of empathy and kindness in the garden of young minds. And a special thank you to our Kickstarter backers. We couldn't have published this book without you!

Jacquelynn-Remery Pearson

Spencer Lee

Laura Lee

Barbara Kotsonis

Bryce Kruchkow for Melissa Hilliker.
"To the love of my life and my inspiration every day."

About the Authors and Illustrator

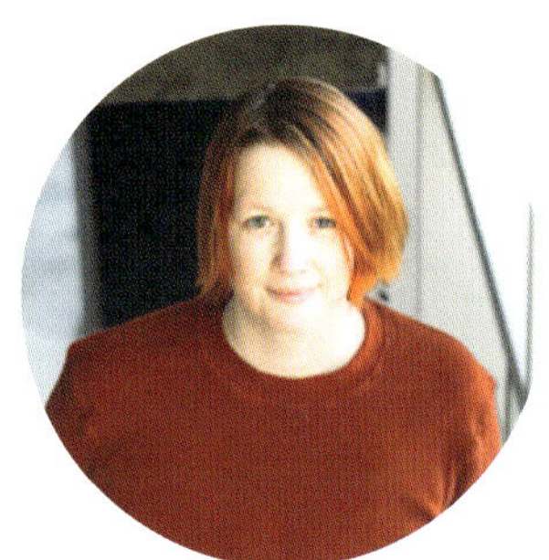

Pey Carter is an author and public speaker specializing in mental health, invisible disabilities, and trauma. Her focus is using storytelling and narrative justice to foster deeper discussions and inspire change. Pey has PTSD, Dysautonomia, Postural Orthostatic Tachycardia Syndrome, Fibromyalgia, Generalized Seizure Disorder, Ehlers-Danlos, Autism, and Avoidance/Restrictive Food Intake Disorder. In her free time, Pey enjoys geocaching and keeping their cat, Bear, from taking over the world.

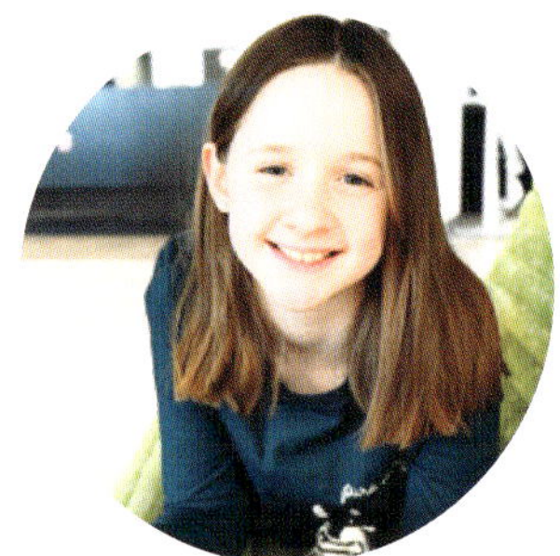

Abigail Bailey is a fun-loving social butterfly who likes to spend time with her friends and family. She is obsessed with anime, especially anything made by Studio Ghibli. Some of her hobbies include biking, playing piano, and singing. One of Abigail's reading goals is to finish the entire Warrior Cat series.

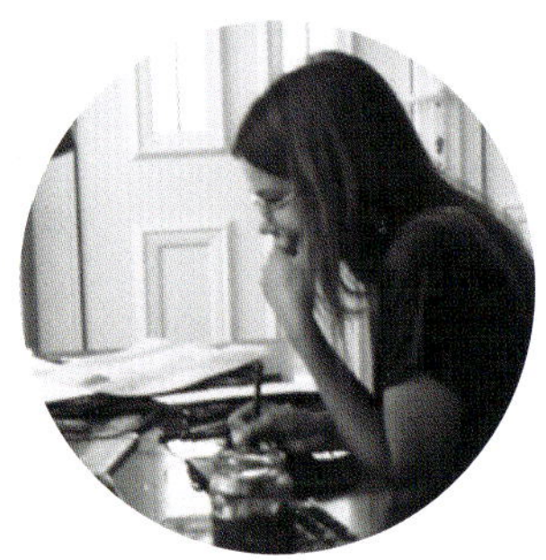

Katarina Stevanović is an artist, educator, and illustrator of over two hundred children's books published across the world. She has a master's degree in the Faculty of Applied Arts from the University of Arts in Belgrade, Serbia, and works in a variety of artistic mediums. In 2021, two books she illustrated–Ni Hao China and Shalom Israel–were recognized by the Story Monster Book Awards.